My Mother, My Son

A true story of love,
determination, and memories...*lost*

Dwayne J. Clark

Also by Dwayne J. Clark: *Help Wanted: Recruiting, Hiring and Retaining Exceptional Staff*

Printed in the United States of America

First Printing, 2012

ISBN 978 0 9848152 0 3

Aegis Living
17602 NE Union Hill
Redmond, Washington 98052

www.MyMotherMySon.com

AUTHOR'S NOTES

I have made every effort to remember names, places, and events accurately, but a few names have been changed when memory didn't serve me or to respect the privacy of those not central to the story of this book. I apologize if your name was forgotten or changed unintentionally.

It is our heartfelt honor to donate all profits of this book to the Alzheimer's Association and the Potato Soup Foundation.

THIS BOOK IS DEDICATED TO MY MOTHER, Mary Colleen Callahan Clark. Most knew her by Colleen, some knew her by Collu, but our family knew her as Mom, Gram, and GG (great-grandmother). She was the freest of free spirits, not wanting to conform to anyone's standards but her own. She had the unique ability to create a vision of her life that was often much better than the reality. She bought fancy clothes when we had no money. She took great trips on a blue-collar salary. She spoke about world events while living in small farm towns. I guess you could say she was a dreamer, but it was a trait that I loved about her.

She was fierce in her love for her children and fierce in her defense of them. She was like a momma bear protecting her cubs. No one came between her and her children. She had a unique sense of self and beauty. She loved sending "beauty shots" of herself. She loved fine clothes and good-looking men. She adored tasty food. She would dance in the living room with no music. Her ultimate day would be surrounded by her children and grandchildren talking about life and the idiosyncrasies of our family. Most who met her loved her from "hello." Her story is not unique to any mother who loves her children. What is unique is the manner in which the universe steered her life's journey.

*"A slip of the tongue is no fault of the mind
and those who mock me are very unkind."*

*"Love all, trust few,
always paddle your own canoe."*

> — Mary Colleen Callahan Clark
> *(Dwayne's mom)*

ACKNOWLEDGEMENTS

I want to thank everyone who spent time working on this book. It was a great effort and a labor of love. I started to write this book nearly five years ago, thinking that I would finish in a year. But as I tracked my mom's decline, the story just kept going. There were so many people who helped me along the way. I am a popcorn-thinker, so I needed people on my team who could organize my thoughts.

To my incredible wife, "T." Thank you for giving me the courage to write this book—even when I doubted myself. Thank you for sharing many laughs and tears on those late nights when I drew upon my memories of Mom. Your support, love, and nurturing are a source of strength for me.

To my siblings, with whom I share this great Mom. Thank you for giving me the space to write this book. I know it was uncomfortable at times and still may be, but you never asked me to stop. My goal was to share our wonderful, zany, obsessive mother with the world. Not because she did incredible things to the world at large, but because her experiences may help thousands of other families coping with memory loss. I want my two sisters, Linda and Edweena, to know how much I admire your courage and the fact that you stayed with our mother until, literally, her last breath. Although I am the author of this book, the two of you are the real heroes.... Thank you.

To the rest of my family: I am sure there will be many occasions to ask, "Why wasn't I mentioned in the book, or why didn't you tell the story about me and Gram when...?" Or you might remember a story I told differently. I know, I know, I know. I only had my perspective to write it from, and I can only hope that you find it worthy.

A gem of a person and a very talented writer, Jim Berry, was the first person I contacted. Jimmy has a wonderful creative side, as well as a tenderness that I thought was needed to take my bungled journals into the beginnings of a book. Jimmy worked side-by-side with me for over a year. He taped things that I said, taking my words and making them better. I was experiencing Mom and her decline in real time so there were days when I would laugh with him and days when I would cry. Jimmy used his incredible talent to launch this book and is responsible for the foundation of the material. Without his tireless effort, this book would never have been written. Thank you, Jimmy, for your incredible writing abilities and friendship.

To my longtime friend David Ford, who is a profound writer himself. He is like the English teacher I hated in school. As a lawyer and a writer, his grammar, editing, and punctuation are impeccable. But more than that, he knows me oh-too-well. He added direction and spice to the book without changing my voice. Thank you, David, for your friendship and support.

To Deborah Sorenson, who helped to pull my thoughts together and redefined the flow of the book. Thank you for the guidance and support during this process.

To Lou Bortone, the man who spent nearly six months with me to guarantee that the book unfolded like I wanted. He brought forth my innermost thoughts and made them make sense. He helped to craft my experiences in an emotional way that created a story for the reader. Thanks Lou, you were great.

To Janet Goldstein, who took the draft version of this book and polished it like a fine gem. She cut and chopped to make it into a worthy book. We spent months together and sometimes worked late into the night to get one paragraph just right. Thanks for your technical competence and incredible writing ability.

To Heather Hayes, who took this book over the finish line. Your attention to every detail and crafting of each sentence was sublime. Every comment and markup was made with thought and care.

To the many others who assisted along the way, thank you:

Jennifer Bartlett

Lynn Behar

Nate Billig

Mardi Boss

Ira Elliott

Doug Griepp

Kim Hall

Connie Jones

Terry Korotzer

Judy Meleliat

Jerry Meyer

Victor Nebre

Norene Ott

Cat Peterson

Lem Putnam

Mark Schneider

Lisa Schuman

Barbara Van Wollner

Diane Warshal

CONTENTS

Part 3. Sailing Away:
The Move 119

Part 4. Being in the Now:
This Is Our Life 183

My Dear Son,

I am so proud of you. You have
_____ so much for so many. Who
_____ have thought that you would
_____ning these awards and
_____ this much success? Well,
_____ld. I always knew that you
_____ make it, son. We had a
_____ time, but you used that hard
_____ as an education to fuel you.
God has given you the chance to
help others and you have seized
the moment. I want you to know
how proud I am of you, how you
have exceeded my expectations, how
you have always been there for me. A
mother could not be more satisfied with
her son. You have done it, you have made
it, you have arrived. I love you so much.

Mom

Mary Colleen Callahan Clark, circa 1967

INTRODUCTION—THE CALL TO HELP

In the year 2000 I began to keep a journal about my mother. She had started to change in ways that were alarming, exhibiting behaviors that, at times, were very different from that of the person I had always known. She could now be moody and short-tempered. She would forget things she shouldn't have forgotten, and she had started drinking.

Even though most of my professional life had been devoted to working with very frail seniors, I didn't want to face the reality that my own Mom was herself getting old and frail. Frail, or dependent, was not who she ever had been, and it's certainly not how I continued to experience her outsized influence and fighting spirit in my own life. From my school days, we were a team of two who fought for our survival. And I still felt like we were that team, that pair of fighters—even if we'd fallen into the trap of distance that so often besets adult relationships.

As Mom's condition worsened, and she ultimately was diagnosed with both Alzheimer's disease and Parkinson's disease, I started writing more and more. Several years into her decline, in a sad irony, my mother became a resident in one of the assisted living communities run by the company I had founded, Aegis Living. My mother, the person who pushed me so hard to achieve worldly success, was now living in the very business I had started as a fulfillment of that shared dream. Our fatherless family had grown up with nothing, yet my larger-than-life mother always believed in me. Even when I went outrageously off track with no indication that I could ever get back on, my mother still called me a "big shot."

So here I was, founder of a company and a CEO. I had made it: I was running a progressive company that was expanding exponentially. Yet my mother was experiencing that success from the inside, as a resident, a completely different vantage point that I would have ever predicted, or wanted.

My key staff and all the people who worked at my mother's Aegis community knew she was in our care. They would ask me how she was doing, but they would also ask after me, sincerely wanting to know how I was holding up. When I told them about my struggles, I sometimes shared a piece of writing from my journal that captured what I was going through. The changes I was witnessing in my mother and the personal challenges I was dealing with were creating new conversations among us. Although I had been doing the larger work of helping the older people in our communities, it was now clear that my heart wasn't fully aware of what true helping meant. I didn't fully understand on a personal level how the services we provided affected a resident on a daily basis—and reverberated throughout that resident's entire family. Indirectly, my experience amplified the work we were doing and how we were doing it.

From these very personal exchanges, some staff and colleagues encouraged me to do two things: First, they suggested that I start writing a blog. Secondly, they urged me to write a book about my experience with my mother and her journey with aging and, eventually, dementia and Parkinson's.

I took up the challenge and began the blog, writing in as personal and vulnerable a way as I could about my feelings, my confusions, even my anger. Then people started writing me. They thanked me for my candor and for sharing my painful experiences in an effort to help others. I heard from family members, experts, and strangers from all walks of life and situations. It became its own community, a small one but caring.

This book turned out to be a natural step in the process. The more I shared and the more I tried to live the philosophy we teach—that every person is a whole human being, that we all have gifts, memories, a legacy, a soul—the more I connected with stories from my mother's colorful (to put it mildly) childhood and motherhood and my own past. I connected more deeply to the memories that have shaped my life and the person I've become. Not all good, to be sure, but mostly.

That knitting together of the long ago, the present, and everything in between makes up the content of this book. Too often when people get sick in this country we refer to them as their disease: The cancer patient or the diabetic. We overlook the richness of experience and personality that underlies that person. We forget their life, their contributions. We forget what lives on in all the people around them. And this is never truer than when facing the reality of memory loss, when a person slowly recedes from the identity they've manifested for so long.

We need an antidote. Our society needs an antidote to this invisibility.

This book makes one life visible. It shares the story of my mother, her inspiration to me, and her legacy of doing things with a flair and determination that left her only at the end. It shares her tireless work ethic, her sense of humor, her feistiness, her sometimes destructive attraction to men. It shows the world who she was beyond her disease. Not because my mother was famous or did anything truly extraordinary to the outside world, but to make sure that she—and the thousands and millions like her—is remembered not just for the ten percent of her life afflicted by memory loss, but for the whole of who she was.

In describing her ten-year-long odyssey with Alzheimer's and interweaving it with the stories and lessons that made up the whole of her life, and mine too, I hope others will take away lessons in how to "do" this passage and to find one's way—in spite of the challenges.

The fact is, with Alzheimer's or dementia, there is no running or hiding. To truly understand these diseases, to truly help in whatever way you are able, you have to understand the loss of who the person was. It is not simply that the disease is devastating; it is the devastation of human life that is left behind.

PROLOGUE—THE LETTER

It was such an emotionally charged night, in many ways the culmination of a long, difficult, fantastic journey. My stomach was doing back flips. My head swirled in a stew of emotions— pride, anxiety, and ironically, some sadness. Sadness because my mother couldn't be here to see this.

Tonight I was being honored with the Lifetime Achievement Award by King County Senior Services, an award given to Seattle leaders in senior services for their contributions in working with the elderly.

The awards ceremony was a formal black-tie affair with over five hundred people in the audience. Of course, my family and friends would be there to support me, but I couldn't help lamenting my mother's absence.

As I finished putting on my tuxedo, I stood facing the mirror to arrange my tie one last time. Out of the corner of my eye, I noticed a small envelope. *Strange,* I thought. *Where did that come from?* Stranger still was the writing. The card was addressed to "My Son, Dwayne." I couldn't make sense of it since my father, who I barely knew, had passed away a few years earlier, and my mother was in no condition to be writing or sending cards.

As I tried to figure out the mystery, I tore open the envelope and found a hand-written letter inside that read:

My Dear Son,

I am so proud of you. You have done so much for so many. Who would of thought that you would be winning these awards and having this much success? Well, I would. I always knew that you would make it, son. We had a hard time, but you used that hard time as an education to fuel you. God has given you the chance to help others and you have seized the moment. I want you to know how proud I am of you, how you have exceeded my expectations, how you have always been there for me. A mother could not be more satisfied with her son. You have done it, you have made it, you have arrived. I love you so much.

Mom

With this letter was a separate note from someone very special to me, Bobbie Berry. Bobbie is like a member of our family and the favorite aunt you always go to for advice. When my wife, Terese, and I were looking to hire someone to help us with entertaining and running our household, Bobbie came highly recommended by a friend who said she was looking to change jobs. When Bobbie arrived for the interview, it turned out that Terese knew her already—she'd been the floral assistant at the shop where Terese first ordered flowers for me when we started dating. We didn't see the sense in interviewing anyone else. We hired her that day and she's been with us for years.

Bobbie's note explained the letter from Mom:

Dwayne,

This letter is not from your mother, it is from me. I wrote it. But I know as a mother that this is what your mother would write. I know as a mother how proud she must be of you—as am I.

Love you,

Bobbie

This was one of the kindest things anyone had ever done for me. Obviously, Bobbie and my family understood that this award was a milestone that I so wished my mother could see. The fact that the woman who made this all possible could not share the moment with me left me feeling empty.

Later, as I nervously prepared to take the stage to accept the award, I surveyed all the people in the audience who were there to support me. Only Mom was missing. I watched as the emcee was about to walk to the podium to introduce me, and then without notice, I saw my family turning toward the wings of the ballroom. Out of the corner of my eye, I saw one of my mother's care managers, Maurice, wheeling her into the ballroom and over to our table at the front of the hall. Despite her condition and her eighty-five years, Mom looked like a movie star.

My entire clan turned to catch my reaction. My son, Adam, looked up and said, "Well Dad, it just wouldn't be right if Gram wasn't here." As I struggled to fight back tears, the emcee introduced me and called me to the podium. I bent down, kissed my mom, and whispered, "Help me hold it together, Mom."

As I began my acceptance speech, I announced that there was only one person who was responsible for my success and for this award: "My mother." I choked up as I pointed to her. The crowd burst into applause. My lips quivered, my voice broke, and although my mother was unaware of her surroundings, I was filled with joy that she could be there.

Part 1.

Daring and Denial:
Mom's Different

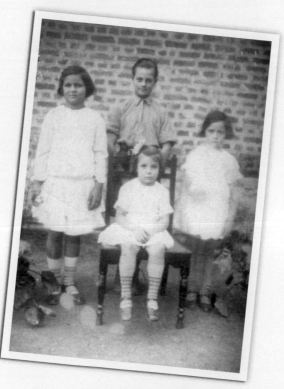

India, circa 1927: Colleen and siblings

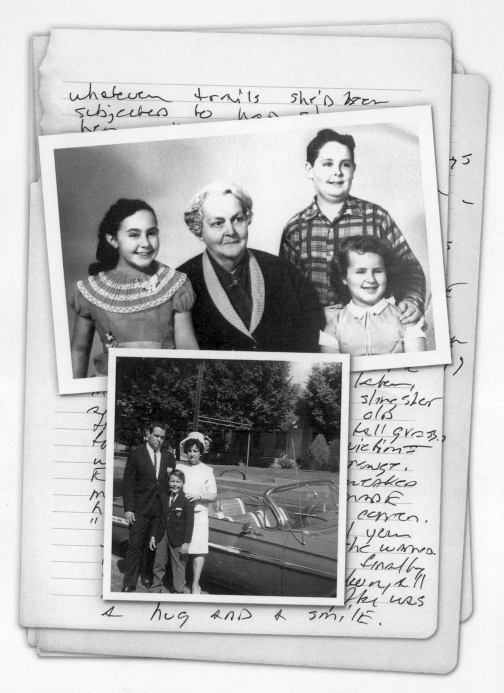

Lewiston, Idaho 1957: Linda Clark Walker, Granny, Larry Clark and Edweena Skinner

Lewiston, Idaho 1967: Larry, Colleen and Dwayne

When the World Made Sense

Alzheimer's is a long and painful path, and there is simply no way of knowing if Mom has a month, a week, or a day. For now, all I can do is sit helplessly at my mother's bedside, watching this cruel disease slowly take her away from everyone she loves and everything she has accomplished in her remarkable life.

On her bedside table is a photograph of us from 1966, when I was seven years old. It's a full head-to-toe view of the both of us, standing next to each other on the sidewalk outside our house in Lewiston, Idaho. Mom has her arm around me and looks a little tired, but she has that trademark grin on her face, while I force a smile and stand at attention. I can still hear her saying, "Stand up straight, my son," with a lilt in her voice, the barest trace of a British accent. That black-and-white image, grainy and slightly out of focus, is a time machine for me. I stare at it and I go back to that place, that tiny house we lived in with my older brother and two sisters and all the drama and strife and love that shook its walls. And then there's today, and where we are now.

My mother is sleeping, a tiny shell of the strong, confident woman she was until only a few years ago. I listen for her breath, a slip of air that seems too thin to sustain life. I find myself inhaling and exhaling to her tempo, almost willing her to keep breathing. I study the lines of her face that track from chin to eye in perfect thin folds, her gaunt cheeks gently puffing. She's so still. Did she stop breathing just then? I wait. She puffs again. And then again. Relief follows a sense that I'm being absurd. I'm so weary of this, wishing it could be any other way than what it is. But there's no escaping or turning back.

Despite Mom's advanced age, I still see her as she was in that picture over forty years ago—glowing, so full of energy, the unpredictable-funny-devoted-sometimes selfish-crazy-beautiful woman she was. I rise to open the curtains and a trace of light falls across her face. She sighs in her sleep.

I have worked in the senior housing field for more than twenty years, and it's as if that period was nothing more than intensive training for this one moment with my mother—but I don't feel prepared. I don't think anyone ever is.

My first position working in elder care had been a literal god-send in a period of professional and personal crisis. Since child-hood, I had wanted to be a criminal lawyer, but that got de-railed midway through college when my girlfriend told me she was pregnant. We got married and I downgraded my dream.

I looked for and found a different position in the criminal justice system, working on a tactical team for the department of corrections and training as a hostage negotiator. The marriage, however, was shaky from the start, and we both knew it was over fifteen months in. We'd had a second child by then, and though we soon divorced, my responsibilities and role as a parent continued.

Fortunately, my job provided financial security, success, and excitement, and I was good at it too, receiving numerous pro-motions from early on. But when I found myself transferred to another local department and trapped working at a prison in a cold, hopeless corner of Washington State, I began doubting everything about myself and my dreams.

It's hard to believe that two conversations could shift the direction my life would take, but they did. The first was seren-dipitous. On a dreary day, one of many during that period of my life, and without really thinking about it, I pulled into the gravel parking lot next to a barely used Catholic church I had passed many times on the stretch of road just outside the nearby town. I had long imagined stopping in, more from a sense of childhood obligation than spiritual belief or need. But the day I finally went in, all I wanted was a quiet place where I could sit and think, a place away from the routines that were eating away at me.

It turned out to be my come-to-God moment—a conversation with Him in which I poured out everything about my situation and my despair with what I was making of my life. I talked about my kids and how I wanted a good environment for them and to be a proper role model, not an angry, frustrated father like my own. I talked about the kind of work I wanted to do, the kind where I would be helping people who wanted and needed it, not monitoring and controlling people trapped in a dark and sinister world separate from everyone else. I even asked God for a job where I could wear a tie to work. Hey, it was my conversation.

Well, God didn't say a thing during that moment, but I received a message. I basically had a choice: I could start acting the way I wanted to act and I could start doing what I wanted to be doing or I could keep doing what I had been doing. The power was within me to live the life I wanted—and I could start right now. I truly believed that this was His message to me, and I knew I had to remake my future one step at a time.

The second conversation was with my sister Linda. One day around that same time, we were talking on the phone and I told her how unhappy I was. I wondered out loud if I had it in me to restart my education and get a law degree. Her quick response completely threw me for a loop. She was running a senior services program in Montana and she actually knew about a position at a senior housing facility. She was adamant that I apply for it. She said it was the "wave of the future." When I gently reminded her that I had no experience whatsoever for the job, she turned the tables on me and asked me point blank if I knew administration, budgeting, activity planning, food service, staff training—a veritable checklist of my current responsibilities, albeit with a different type of resident. The only thing I lacked was experience in sales and marketing.

Though it seemed like a crazy idea, I researched the field and the company, and with no other options in sight, I applied for and got the job. They started me a notch or two below the level they'd been recruiting for so I could prove myself. I was all of twenty-six years old, but within a couple of years I had shown what I could do. I became a troubleshooter for the company and moved up to a manager role.

Those pleading prayers to God on a rainy afternoon had been answered. I had found a field where I could truly help people and thrive professionally at the same time. I had set in motion choices that led me on a new, more fulfilling life path.

Year after year, my mother faithfully followed my career, cheering me on when I started in that first job in assisted living and rooting for me through all my promotions, moves, and company changes. She was my biggest cheerleader. When I made the leap to start Aegis Living and test my own ideas and ambitions for elder care from the ground up, Mom would visit me wherever I was based, taking interest in all the places and people involved. When she was nearly eighty years old, she visited an Aegis community and played bingo, commenting on how "cute" all those old people were—as if that life stage was still years off for her.

She never thought of herself as old and she *never* told people her age. She'd color her hair and she'd tell people it was natural. Youth was her friend, her identity.

As my mother crept into her eighties, however, her memory started to slip. First, little things were lost in time; then the memory gaps become more significant. She couldn't possibly have Alzheimer's, I'd say to myself—she still had black hair and joked with us about finding the right man.

If anyone would know whether my mother had this disease, it would be me. Yet I remained skeptical and resistant, as did my siblings. At each stage of her decline, I fought or denied the new reality: the diagnosis itself, the need for help, and the decision to move her to assisted living.

But here we were. Her first weeks at Aegis, and she seemed so weak and so far away. How quickly the last crises piled up. How shocking that we'd denied how much help she needed. The feelings of guilt and abandonment were beyond extreme.

We tried to look on the bright side of life. We'd remind each other how much we had to be thankful for—family, friends, work, prosperity, our own health. We tried to maintain that state of being, counting our many blessings, but my mother's condition would hang over us like an endless dark cloud. This was our mother, and she was being taken away from us, not all at once, but slowly and cruelly, a little bit more day by day.

As I sat back down in my mother's room, watching her sleep, I tried to recall all of my own blessings. I remembered when I was a boy how close Mom and I became after my brother and two sisters left the house to get married and start their own lives. She treated me like a friend as well as a young son. We became inseparable, and at night, as I'd drift off to sleep, it wasn't unusual for me to be gripped by a deep fear that I would wake up to find Mom dead. I prayed every night for God to keep her with me. Now, so much time had gone by and so many miles had been traveled. I wanted to tell her that we had made it, that we're still here. But that's not quite true, is it? We're not both here.

I checked her again, lying so still, and found her breathing even shallower than before. I remember doing this with my kids when they were babies, repeatedly going in to make sure they were still warm, breathing, alive. I bet Mom did that for me, too. Now I was doing it for her. I wanted to shake her until she woke so I could tell her, "I love you," and "You were a good mom—no, a great one." But I let her sleep, imagining that her dreams are kinder than her waking life, where she spends so much of her time disoriented, scared, and sick.

As I sat there, watching over the living remains of my mother, I saw that there is a lesson to be learned. A lesson that proclaims, once and for all, that we must live here and now, in this moment, and we must find a way to cherish it, even as it slips away and changes again into something new.

A conversation in the hallway interrupted my thoughts, reminding me that it's time to make that awkward transition that happens at the end of each visit: In this room, I am the son of a resident in a memory-care unit at an assisted living community. Out there, among the staff members that take such good care of her, I am the chief executive officer of the company that operates the community, pays their salaries. I know there will have been at least a little buzz about "the boss" being in the building. I guiltily wondered whether they think I visit Mom often enough.

I glanced once more at that old, grainy photo of Mom and me back then. There are moments when I have imagined stepping through that picture and traveling back to a time when so much was still ahead of her—and us.

DELHI BEGINNINGS

My mother, Mary Colleen Callahan, was born in India on May 28, 1923, shortly after her parents, Dennis and Agnes, and their brood of children had settled in Delhi so her father could take an executive position with the British Railroad. According to my mother, Dennis Callahan was responsible for scheduling the routes for the entire country's small-gauge commuter rails, a massive job requiring a large crew of traffic controllers. He typically worked ten-hour days, six days a week. But he was rewarded handsomely for his efforts. My mother grew up in a sprawling, fully staffed, fourteen-room mansion with a separate building housing the kitchen in the backyard. The estate overlooked a great grassy slope and faced north and west, toward England. My grandmother, Agnes, dutifully raised her large family in this grand setting while my grandfather served the British Empire.

Colleen (from birth my mom was called by her middle name) was a tiny newborn, and for several days, her survival was in question. My grandmother had already suffered two stillbirths prior to becoming pregnant with my mother, and so the entire household was in a state of high anxiety. As her tiny daughter fought for breath, Agnes lit candles, prayed to St. Brigid, protector of newborn babies, and never left her side. The family, including all the brothers and sisters, along with a staff of a dozen Indian servants, gathered around the crib at the end of each day to join in the vigil. The servants had difficulty pronouncing my mother's name so they shortened it to Collu, a nickname that stuck. With all that loving attention and perhaps with the invoking of the gods, after four days, baby Collu became ravenously hungry, and after another two days of nearly nonstop feedings, she was alert and happy.

My mother quickly grew to be a loud, fearless, thrill-seeking toddler, and her lust for adventure marked her school years. She was often bored as a student, and much preferred the enticements of the outdoors to math problems and reading lessons.

She loved to tell the stories of the weddings she went to as a little girl and how the women wore the most beautiful silk saris, long, intricate earrings, and ornate headdresses that rounded to a peak like the towers of the Taj Mahal. The family received invitations to many arts performances, and although her siblings often begged out, my mom was always eager to attend. It could be a theater performance, a musical soiree, or a dance recital. She took in everything her life in India had to offer. She befriended the children of the house servants at an early age, becoming fluent in Hindi—and she remembered many phrases well into her eighties.

My mother was an equal-opportunity aficionado of all things India. She especially loved the outdoors, the wildlife, the monkeys that lived in the trees in the backyard, and the family of gazelles that marched across the grass not thirty feet away from the porch where she and her siblings spent time in the evenings and listened to the tigers roaring in the distance.

Still, home wasn't always a playground, not with a mother like Agnes, a patron of discipline who stood an imposing five-foot-ten and tipped the scales at nearly 180 pounds. My grandmother, "Granny" to me, was a shrewd woman who'd survived a brutal childhood as an orphan in England's Irish-Catholic foster care system. Her own mother had died in childbirth and her father, a traveling showman who had shared dates with Wild Bill Hickok, was so stricken with grief that he abandoned her just a few weeks after she was born. Except for the occasional postcard, my grandmother never heard from her father again. She rarely spoke of her childhood, but clearly, whatever trials she'd been subjected to had sharpened her will to a fine point. She was strength and control personified. And then there was my mother, a hellraiser without peer, her own mother's complete opposite.

My mom was an ace with a slingshot and often sniped servants and passersby with pebbles. Once, she hit a servant in the head and opened a cut in his scalp. Granny tracked her down, found the slingshot, and burned it in front of her, making her promise to never do it again. A week later, my mom had a new slingshot and was back to her old tricks, hiding in the tall grass for any unsuspecting victim who might come into range.

Exasperated, Granny tweaked my mom's ear and made her stand in a corner. "You just wait until your father comes home," she warned.

When my grandfather finally came through the door, though, all he had for his daughter was a smile and a hug. She was far and away his favorite and my mom adored him right back. As she got older, on her breaks from private school in the mountains north of Delhi, Mom often worked for him as a personal assistant. He entrusted her with receipts and payroll checks that she would run, literally, to the bank. At noon, they would eat lunch together and at the end of the day they stood side by side, as each rail worker filed by the sign-out sheet. Many of them couldn't write their names so they'd dab their thumbs in black ink and leave a print as their unique signature.

At home, dinners were candle-lit affairs with linen napkins and heavy silverware, promptly served at 9 p.m. by a team of servants. Table manners were as important as the food itself. No slouching was allowed. The girls sat on the edge of their chairs with straight backs, and under no circumstances were they allowed to rest their elbows on the table. They would be served course after course of soups, curries, and fancy rice dishes with all kinds of vegetables, nuts, and spices. The control Granny taught her children continued to the last moment. No matter how delicious the food, they had to follow the Indian custom of leaving a little behind on the plate to convey to the host (in this case their mother and the servants) that the hospitality was plentiful and appreciated.

After dinner the mood changed. The family engaged in reading, card games, storytelling, and singing. My mother would even perform little *a cappella* solos for her siblings. And then it was bedtime. If he was home, my grandfather would check in with each child, and he always saved the youngest, my mom, for last. She had one of the biggest bedrooms in the house all to herself, and her father had even indulged her with a custom king-sized bed made from the wood of a Banyan tree. He would tuck her in and read her a story before turning out the light and closing the door.

During these India-saturated growing-up years my mother knew that she mattered and believed that she was destined for good—if not great—things. When events soon chased her to America and dramatically altered her future, she never lost her childhood sense of ambition. In spite of her radically changed circumstances, she imparted her dreams and expectations to her children, especially me—the youngest in her brood.

SHOES TO FILL: "YOU'RE A BIG SHOT"

I imagined my mother's exotic and exciting childhood in India as some kind of wondrous fairy tale. When I was young I would often ask her to retell my favorite stories.

"Did you really ride your elephant to school?" I'd ask.

"Yes, on occasion. Father frowned upon it, but I could usually get away with it once in a while."

I knew even then that my mother loved to make a grand entrance, whether as a schoolgirl on an elephant or as an adult wearing a party dress she couldn't afford.

"What was the elephant's name?"

She'd laughed loudly. Her strong laugh was one of her trademarks, ever present.

"Oh, my son. There were many elephants on the property—to do all of the heavy lifting. I rarely rode the same one twice. I'm not sure they even had names."

I had heard many details of the fine furnishings, fancy clothes, and tutors, so it didn't surprise me that there would have been a lot of elephants on call too.

I would press her to say something to me in Hindi, and she'd respond with a string of syllables like "Apa eka bara soa punah..."

"What does that mean?" I would ask in awe, always amazed that she spoke such a strange and musical language. On more than one occasion the answer was: "I said, 'You are a big shot!'" It was one of the regular refrains she'd toss out to me, always with a trace of the English accent, so it made sense that it was something that she heard and knew in Hindi as well.

When she came to the United States as a young war bride, her fortunes had changed dramatically. Having such a privileged beginning to her life, though, seemed to inspire her to believe that great things were in store for us children as well. She grew up with a big elephant and a big mansion; we grew up with little more than big dreams.

HIDING UNDER THE GREEN CHAIR

In stark contrast to my mother, who was so close to her father—a man who managed to make time to develop a close
relationship with all of his children—my dad was out of my life
before I reached first grade.

When my mom discovered my dad was cheating on her, she
took it as a sign that it was time to move on and we never really
looked back. She picked up and moved us four kids and herself
into a little house on Eleventh Avenue in Lewiston, Idaho, a
small paper-mill town in the elbow formed by the Snake and
Clearwater Rivers. The only thing that made Lewiston feel
bigger was Clarkston, its smaller twin on the other side of the
Snake in Washington State. It still amuses me to think of the
rivalries between these towns named after the famous explorers
who charted a path to the Pacific. They were both filled with
cowboys and pickup trucks, regardless of which bank of the
river you were on.

I was seven or eight years old when we left behind the family
ranch in Riggins, Idaho. More significantly, we left behind my
dad. It was the last of a series of moves for me, my mother, my
brother Larry Ray, my sisters, Linda Kay and Edweena Fay, and
of course, our wiener dog, Herman May. (Yes, even Herman
hadn't escaped the middle name rhyming madness, nor had I.
My name is Dwayne Jay.)

My father was a startlingly smart man with a high degree of
curiosity, and things just didn't hold his interest for very long.

In fact, my mom said the Army had tested his IQ and determined that he was a genius. The few times I saw him as an adult, he always found a way to mention those tests and flaunt this bit of status.

Our restless dad took turns as a plumber, electrician, farmer, ranch hand, and auctioneer, and he had served as chairman of the local Chamber of Commerce.

We were fortunate that family life also failed to hold his interest, though I'm sure it didn't feel that way to my mother at the time. I remembered him as stern, indifferent, or altogether absent, except when he was just mean. His explosions of fury still punctuate my memories like firecrackers. He seemed to believe that cruelty was part of what it meant to be a man. (When he reappeared in my life in my forties, his behavior only reaffirmed my childhood image. Oddly, I was just a bit grateful to him, since he validated what might have seemed like stories whose ugliness had become exaggerated over time.)

One of my earliest memories is a testament to my father's rage. I was five and asleep in my bedroom when the yelling started.

"Who does she think she is, defying *my* rules in *my* house?" my father spewed. My mother's voice was higher pitched than usual, but trying to sound calm, she replied: "Ed, don't do this. She's not that late."

"Look at her walking up like she owns the place," Dad bellowed as he watched my sister coming home late from a date she wasn't supposed to be on in the first place. I slid out of bed and quietly peeked out from my bedroom. I could imagine my sister looking pleased as she returned from her date, wholly unprepared for what awaited her. I'd seen that look before. I wished I could warn her away from opening the front door.

I crept down the hall even though I'd get in trouble for being out of bed. Fear pulled me toward the scene. As soon as I got to the living room, I realized I had made a terrible mistake. My father's anger was palpable.

My sister pushed open the door with a big grin on her face, nearly bumping into my father before she realized he was there. Now she looked as frightened as I felt, but she tried to sidestep him as if he were only an inconvenience. He grabbed her arm as he slammed the door shut with his foot and twisted her around to face him.

I scrambled behind, and then under, the green living room chair that was closest to the hallway. He had taken off his belt and palmed the massive steel buckle with its insignia of a bronco in mid-buck and wrapped the thick, worn leather around his knuckles. He raised his arm and slapped my sister's face with the back of his hand, knocking her to the floor. She looked more stunned than hurt and slowly got to her hands and knees. But Dad wasn't finished. He uncoiled the belt from his fist and began to whip her backside with it.

Mom jumped to protect her daughter, yelling, "Stop, Ed! For God's sake, stop!" But there was no stopping him. My father pushed my mother to the ground next to my sister and began to flail at both of them, as if they were a team of mules that had refused to pull his wagon.

I cowered from the safety of the green chair with its mahogany legs, the cane weaving of the seat forming my own little shelter. I desperately wanted to run out and stop my father, but terror pinned me under the chair. I huddled there in my pajamas, shaking, the rough caning scratching my head as I followed the length of leather, rising and falling. My mother and sister clung to each other, sharing the beating, hardly making a noise except for short, sharp sobs of grief and pain. Mom tried to shelter my sister's back from the brunt of the attack.

I think fatigue was the only thing that stopped my father's rage. He finally looked down and shouted, "Shut up, the both of you!" Despite the harshness of the words, his voice was emotionless. Then he looked around, almost startled, his eyes surveying the room as if he were trying to figure out where he was. I tried to shrink further underneath the chair, but the motion caught his attention. I was sure it was my turn for a beating. My father saw the fear on my face and I saw the power in him fade away as he turned, strode across the room, and without another word, slammed the front door behind him.

The two days before he returned home were, in equal measures, calm and tense. We were glad he was gone, sorry he was gone, ashamed for ourselves and for him. I guess it's not surprising, then, that no one ever mentioned what had happened.

Divorce was inevitable for my parents, even in those conservative times in rural Idaho. Shortly after that horrible night, my mother found out that my father was cheating on her. Someone she knew had seen him with a waitress in Spokane. With dramatic flair and her emotions running high, she got in the car, drove the four-and-a-half hours to the big city, and actually found him with his mistress.

There was no way she could take him back, not with his abuse and now his lying, and she knew he didn't want to come back anyway. Granny came to live with us to help after the divorce, Mom and us kids moved shortly after, and my dad just disappeared. He didn't say goodbye, he didn't visit, and he didn't pay child support. In a way he became a ghost, an imaginary presence on to which I could project my ideals of what I wanted my father to be.

Mom embraced her new life as the head of the family, but it was immensely difficult. She had come to America as the wife of Ed Clark, an American G.I. stationed in India just before that vast country attained independence, and that life had now disintegrated. Suddenly husbandless, she was branded with the scarlet letter of "D": divorcée.

CELEBRATING AND WORRYING

The party took months to plan and just a few moments for it
to fall apart. Celebrating my 40th birthday and marking all the
good in my life meant so much to me. I was still married to my
second wife, though we knew this was sort of the end. I had
dedicated my life to improving myself, raising my children, and
building a company that mattered.

This landmark birthday party, though, wasn't about regrets. It
was a moment to savor all that was right. The house sparkled.
The living room had been converted into a dance hall, and we
set up a cigar tent in the backyard. There were lighted paths so
guests could easily come outside and enjoy the night air. The
late autumn nights were getting chilly, but it was a clear evening.
Perfect.

All kinds of delicious, indecently rich party food was spread out
on tables everywhere: fried chicken, barbecued pork ribs, Swed-
ish meatballs, potato skins, nachos, various dips, and cupcakes
with creamy frosting in every color and flavor imaginable. It
was a night to indulge myself and everyone else.

I had planned a guest list of about one hundred. Both of my children were there. There were people I had worked with at Aegis
since our founding. Of course, my sisters, Edweena and Linda,
and their children all came, plus dear friends from all parts of my
life who had traveled from states far and wide, many of whom
I hadn't seen in years. I was so touched and proud of the deep
connections I'd made in my life, and I was especially happy that
my mom could also be there to celebrate with me.

I guess it's true for most of us that, even as adults, we want more than anything to get our parents' blessing and approval. In my case, Mom had stuck with me and believed in me through one milestone after another, and many of her dreams for me were finally coming true.

Tonight she arrived with Jack, her latest boyfriend. I'd be the first to admit that I didn't much like him and my sisters didn't either. My mother's choice in men has often been a mystery to me, but Jack was worse than most. A few months before, my mom had watched an "Oprah" show about online dating and, though she'd never before used a computer, decided it was worth a try. She enlisted my sister to help, and within three days, my mother was chatting online with Jack, who had posted a profile along with a picture. "He'll do," my mother had joked.

Edweena set her up with email and instant messenger accounts, and the two love birds were soon communicating two or three times a day.

At first, my mother expected the computer to work just like a phone. Apparently, it was a hoot to see her talking back at the computer as if Jack was on the other end of the line. She'd see Jack's screen name—BIGJACK129—and then his message would appear on the screen accompanied by the soft bloop-bloop sound.

Edweena would read his words aloud to Mom: "Hi, Hon, how are you?"

Mom would then lean into the computer and yell: "I'm good, honey! What's new with you?"

"He can't hear you, Mom," Edweena would try to explain. "It's an instant message." But Mom would only shout louder, as if the problem was simply that Jack couldn't quite catch what she was saying.

Of course, Mom lied about her age immediately, telling her cyber-beau that she was ten years younger, knowing she could pull it off with her hair dyed jet black. He told her he loved her before he even laid eyes on her, and she began calling him her boyfriend.

Jack was a cowboy who styled himself after Johnny Cash. He wore polished black cowboy boots, black pants, black Western shirts with pearl buttons, sunglasses—the whole nine yards. His thick, waxed moustache was perfectly shaped, with the ends curled into points. He was quite a character and energetic for his age, but even so, he could barely keep up with my mom. He was ten years younger, but he looked older, with a shock of gray hair and deep, hard lines carved into his cheeks. He had worked on the Alaskan pipeline for years and was fond of telling stories about his time in the tundra, hunkered down in temperatures of thirty below zero. Rounding out his rough-hewn persona, Jack had been a lifelong drinker and didn't mind sharing his love and need for liquor with anyone within earshot. He liked to joke that when he wanted to take it easy, he'd switch from whiskey to vodka.

My problem with Jack the few times I'd met him wasn't that he was a big talker. I had gotten used to that quality in my mom's boyfriends a long time ago. Or even that he was a big drinker, because that wasn't new either. It was because this time, for some reason, Mom was drinking right alongside him. And that wasn't like her. She'd always been a party girl, and she still loved a night out, but alcohol wasn't involved in the attraction. She just liked the social scene.

Now, though, it seemed like she had a drink in her hand every time I visited, no matter what our plans or activities. It was nothing for her to put down four or five big vodkas in short or-der, and it showed. It would have to: She was pickling her brain. One day, Edweena sat on the sofa and felt a lump under her hip.

She pulled out an empty vodka bottle. Because Edweena shared her little house with our mother, she was the one who was confronted with this new phase in Mom's life. Though Edweena was always loath to complain, or even mention what was going on, I could tell it was starting to drive her crazy.

Thus, when my mother and Jack arrived for my birthday celebration, it was such a relief to see her beaming, beautiful, composed, and sober.

She wore a new outfit: white wool slacks and a red blazer set off with a pearl choker. At 75, she still knew how to make a grand entrance. Seeing her so happy and confident made me relax and feel suddenly complete, as if my world had come full circle and we were all exactly where we were supposed to be. It was easy to put aside the concerns about my mom that had started to trouble me more.

"Oh, Dwayne," my mother exclaimed, hugging me exuberantly as she walked in. "Look at your home! Look at all this! It's just beautiful." She made her way into the living room with Jack and took on the role of the grand dame and proud matriarch. It was hard to tell whose celebration it was. Watching her smile and hold court at my party filled me with happiness.

For hours, I mingled with the crowd, catching up with old friends. Music filled the house and set the tone, mixing just the right amount of old classics with current hits and tempting me over and over again to jump onto the dance floor—first with my daughter and then old college friends and current colleagues.

Before the evening was out, I made sure I visited the cigar tent for a brandy and an opportunity to reminisce. I found some buddies with their feet up, sharing stories that always seemed to get better with age.

In the cool night air, the house glowed like a jewel. As I headed back to the party, I could almost imagine my mom as a girl long ago growing up in India. Had I planned the outdoor tent to bring back the sense of exotic romance that my mom transferred to my own childhood?

I had just come through the front door and was almost to the dance floor when Katie, one of the young Aegis staff members attending the party, came running up to me. "Umm, I think your mom just punched my friend," she whispered, looking embarrassed and confused.

I rushed to the scene beside the dance floor.

Edweena was already there. She had grabbed our mother under her arms and was dragging her to the den while Mom yelled and cursed, seemingly possessed. I was still trying to process what was unfolding. As I followed them into the room, I looked back and saw that Jack still stood near Julia, Mom's victim, a concerned look on his face. Apparently, Jack had been dancing with Julia, and Mom had decked her out of jealousy. Julia looked so young and vulnerable, trying to figure out what had just happened. The forty-year age difference seemed particularly glaring.

"What the hell do you think you're doing?" I demanded of my mother as soon as the den door slammed behind me. "That's it, Mom. If you can't control your drinking in my house, then you need to leave."

"Oh, Dwayne," she said, attempting to sound reasonable and desperate to cover up the mess she had made. But she was slurring her words. "It wasn't that bad. Your sister likes to make a big deal of things. You're both overreacting."

"You can't be serious!" I shouted. "I don't even know that poor girl you just punched. Mom, this is humiliating—for both of us."

She refused, or at least pretended not, to understand why she had to go home early. I felt bad for Edweena whose night was cut short too, as she was tasked with getting Mom back to Jack's and into bed.

I rejoined the guests, made apologies, and tried to enjoy what was left of the festive night.

But I knew something was missing. It wasn't the mother Edweena had hurried out the door—she was the last person I wanted around right now—rather it was the mother who I thought had arrived a couple of hours earlier, the mother who'd been by my side through thick and thin. She had shown up tonight as the belle of the ball, but had to be led out like some kind of drunken female cowboy who had just busted up the saloon. The person I missed was the younger mom, the glamorous, supportive, sometimes outlandish mom from my childhood and early adulthood. Not the loose cannon she was becoming. As I watched the night begin to fall on my 40th birthday, a thought flickered through my mind: *I'm too young for my mom to get old.*

INCORRIGIBLE

Mom was always feisty—no question about that. But there was a clear difference between the mischievous spirit that Mom had always pushed to the limit and the edge that was starting to tinge her colorful personality. In her younger days, Mom's main foils were the Catholic nuns at boarding school.

From the age of six years old until she graduated at fifteen, Mom attended St. Mary's Parochial in Nainital, India, in the foothills of the Himalayas. The school was a destination for many of the well-heeled European girls in India. She and my grandfather would make the all-day trip by train north from Delhi. Given her father's position with the British Railway, the two of them would be treated like royalty. At the end of the line, a team of Sherpas would escort them the rest of the way along a steep, snowy trail that ended at the gate of the all-girl's boarding school.

My mom never forgot the first time she arrived at St. Mary's. She was awed by the Gothic school buildings, monastery, and cathedral, all set against a backdrop of billowing clouds and jutting peaks. The British nuns who ran the school were equally imposing, she said, dressed in identical, pristine white habits.

The nuns sounded a gong when it was time for visitors to leave. When my mother realized that her father was going, she burst into tears and clung to him, begging him to take her back.

But of course that was not to be. He dabbed her wet face with his handkerchief and then handed it to her. "You keep this with you," she remembered him saying. "It will remind you of home."

St. Mary's proved an incredibly strict and unforgiving environment. Studies were rigorous, and punishments were quickly dispensed for any infraction. My mother tried to abide by the rules, but no matter how good her posture and how hard she studied, she couldn't refrain from misadventure for long. Her desire to upend the status quo landed her in constant trouble and her clandestine pranks became legendary.

Once, she intentionally poured black ink on a nun's chair just before a lesson began. When the nun, dressed in her all-white habit, sat down in the puddle of black liquid and then stood again, the class erupted with laughter. She repeated the stunt twice more and would have tried it a fourth time, but one of the other girls tattled. As punishment, my incorrigible mother was forced to kneel in front of a candle for hours, praying for forgiveness. Only after her knees went numb and she crumpled to the floor did the nuns allow her to rejoin her class.

Another time, on a dare, she banged the gong used only by the nuns to signal meals, visitors, and nighttime emergencies. She didn't get caught at first so she kept it up, challenging the nuns to figure out who was doing it and why. Again, a tattletale fingered my mother, and when she was finally caught in the act, the nuns brought out the "Chocolate Stick," a thin cane made of dark, gnarled wood that they reserved for their strictest punishments. They switched her knuckles until welts rose and bruises colored, and when they were done, my mother promised never to do it again. And didn't. Instead, she invented a new scheme whenever the urge to rebel grew too strong.

She loved to recount these accounts of defiance to me as I was growing up. There were occasions when she simply refused to do her school work; instances when she openly challenged the nuns on a point of scripture that didn't make sense to her; and times when she refused to sit still and be quiet just to prove that she wasn't easily bossed around. One of the stories that made the biggest mark on me was when she jumped the wall to visit the nearby Catholic boys' academy in search of companionship and chocolate bars. Always, though, there were punishments, usually in the form of prostration or the Chocolate Stick.

Not surprisingly, my mother was singled out as a troublemaker and became an easy target for the nuns, even if she wasn't always the culprit. They were never able break her will, though. That effort would prove futile with the irrepressible Mary Colleen Callahan.

I was never quite sure what lessons my mother hoped to impart with these stories she'd regale me with as I was growing up. Was she trying to encourage my own daring and rebellion—like mother, like son? Or did she want to remind me—and herself— of her potential for dramatic and courageous (if misguided) acts? It was as if she spent her whole life proving that her independence was justified—necessary, even—and that my knowing about it would somehow serve me well.

YOU AND ME AGAINST THE WORLD

For three years after Mom's divorce, the family—my mother, four children, and Granny—lived in a tiny, crowded, two-bedroom house. There must have been a constant line to use its only bathroom. Larry, twelve years older than me, was taking courses at college but still lived at home. Mom made sure he stayed close by as long as she could. It was easy for me to look up to him, literally and figuratively. He was tall and stocky, and in high school, he was well liked by his classmates, a top student, and clever and quick-witted. He had an entrepreneurial spirit from an early age, and I suppose that may have been the one inheritance we both have acknowledged receiving from our father. Unlike our dad, however, Larry was patient and caring. Everyone called him "Hoss," after the character in the popular western series "Bonanza."

Linda, the fashion queen of the family and just eighteen months younger than Larry, looked like Marlo Thomas in her "That Girl" phase. Fortunately, she was smarter than the TV character and sharper tongued, too. She was so popular that she'd been engaged three times by the time she finished high school.

With the two oldest siblings pretty much out in the world, fifteen-year-old Edweena (who I often referred to as "Dweena") was left to put up with her little brother, who wouldn't leave her girlfriends alone. She was the wild teenager among us, blessed with my mother's prankster spirit and a compassionate heart. I wanted so badly to be part of the teen life that I'd nag and beg to be taken along. "Mom, Dweena won't let me go with her to the Arctic Circle," I'd whine, praying I'd get to tag along when she and her friends went to the local drive-in restaurant, a popular hangout.

"Edweena. Who says you can go to the Arctic Circle?" And Mom would force her to take me or be left behind herself.

"Mo-om!" my sister would plead. "It's Saturday afternoon, and I already did my homework. The other girls' moms all said it's okay."

"Good. Then it's easy enough to take your brother along, or you can stay here with Dwayne and your friends can come over."

Edweena would almost always relent, but with one condition, "Tell him to stop trying to kiss my friends! It's creepy."

My mother would laugh. "Nothing creepy about it. He's a man. That's what men do. Good for you, my son!" She winked at me. It was one of the first of many encouragements I would receive from my mother to be a man—a "real man" by her definition. Despite the abuse she'd received from my father, my mother admired men and deferred to them. That attitude stemmed partly from the culture of her generation and partly from her upbringing, but I would learn soon enough how much she would expect of me as the man of the house. In her own way, she was preparing me for the challenge.

My father's disappearance meant that my mother had to learn quickly how to earn a living and maintain a household. She found a job as the salad girl at the Lewiston Elks Lodge. It paid $1.15 an hour, but she soon figured out that the cook at the club was paid a lot more and was, in some ways, the center of that small universe. Always resourceful, Mom willingly took on someone else's shift whenever asked, especially if it gave her the chance to watch what the cook was doing. Within the year, she was running the kitchen.

Whenever my siblings and I talk about those first years in Lewiston, I recognize just how difficult a time it was. We had no money; Larry, Linda, and Edweena worked odd jobs to help keep the utilities on and to cover their own necessities. Our mother put in long hours and wore herself down just so that we could get by. Yet get by we did, and we have happy memories of the time. We didn't see ourselves as victims, didn't think of ourselves as poor. After all, we had each other. That's what Mom always said, and what she demanded of us, too.

I was happy to go along with our tight-knit ways. As the baby of the family, I enjoyed whatever attention I could get. My siblings, on the other hand, were chomping at the bit and pulling away. Mom would use guilt, genuine need, and love to keep the other ones close by. But in spite of her manipulations, within one six-month period in 1969, all three of my siblings got married in grand weddings and set out to begin their new lives.

With my siblings gone, my mother clung to me as if I were an inoculation against loss. One day I walked into her room and found her crying. As I started to back out of the doorway, she looked right at me and said, "Promise me you'll never leave me, my son. You won't leave me, will you?" I suppose a ten-year-old couldn't see beyond a life with his mother, and that was certainly the case for me, so I was being completely sincere when I stated, "No. I'll never leave you, Mom." I sat on the floor beside her, put my arm around her shoulders, and hugged her.

From that day on, I could no longer say goodbye to my mother, even if I was just heading off to school in the morning. Mom would stand in the front window watching me walk across the yard. My duty was to turn and look back at her so that she could sign "I love you"—a fist against her chest, with thumb, index finger, and pinky extended out. I would make the same gesture, then turn back toward the road, ready to get where I was going. She was my mother and she loved me. But there was more to it than motherly love. Her fears for herself were in play, too: *What if he doesn't come back? What will I do then?*

Occasional nights out—whenever we could afford it—became our special "dates" where I would learn Mom's life lessons and her big plans for my future.

Over a dinner of our favorites, which we came to call "Tasty Food"—for me, a junior burger and fries, and for Mom, a chicken fried steak with a salad buried in Thousand Island dressing so that whatever inherent health value was eradicated—my mother would plot my future. She'd expound on my future as a lawyer, U.S. president, or whatever job title signified to her the greatest achievement of the moment. She seemed to have infinite ambition for me, perhaps because she had so many more years to focus her attention on developing my attributes and potential. In her eyes, it was only a matter of when and how I achieved greatness, never if. The details, of course, were left to me.

She'd often remark that our family was every bit as good and capable as were the Kennedys. President John F. Kennedy had been her hero and her touchstone of success. He was assassinated on the same day as my fifth birthday, November 22, 1963. When I got home from school I found my mom sobbing on the couch. I was so mad at her for being upset on my special day. Then I heard her explain that something was wrong with the president. My birthday party was canceled, forever linking my life with his, along with millions of others who felt touched by his legacy.

Years later, I took that connection to a whole new level and began collecting Kennedy memorabilia—a passion that led to owning the actual Camelot board game that John and Robert played together when they were children.

My mom regularly drilled me on the ways of the world, inculcating me early in her rules to live by:

"Be a gentleman with women."

"You play, you pay."(It would be a few years before I understood that one.)

"Look people in the eye when you have something to say."

"A nice, firm handshake is the key to good business."

Whenever my mother introduced me to someone new, often at the grocery store, I would startle adults who were not used to a child initiating a grown-up handshake.

Most important of all of her lessons: "Love all, trust few, always paddle your own canoe."

There would be other lessons added over the years—her willing me to make up for what she hadn't been able to give me. But there was one lesson that was intended to remain a secret, a covenant, just between the two of us. She'd often whisper it to me when we were alone:

"My son?"

"Yes, my mother."

"It's you and me, kid," she'd state. And then a second time in case there was any doubt: "*You*"—pointing a finger at me—"and *me*"—pointing at herself—"against the world."

"Yes, my mother," I responded dutifully, a little softer this time.

I was her little man being prepared to take on whatever rights and duties fell to the man of the house. It truly was Mom and me against the world.

ART, THE TRAVELING SALESMAN

My secure little world began to show cracks. While my mother worked very hard to provide for us, she was also young enough, vain enough, and desirous enough to be distracted by her own interests.

A couple of times a week, sometimes with girlfriends, more often with men she'd met at the Elks Lodge, Mom would enjoy a night out on the town. Of course, I didn't like any of the guys who came to pick her up and I'd try to get her to come home early. "Be home by eleven," I'd demand, negotiating a curfew for my mom that felt acceptable to me.

"No, that's too early," Mom would argue. "That's just when things get fun!"

"Then definitely by midnight," I'd counter.

When midnight came, as it usually did with no sign of my mother, I would start to worry and would track her down all over town.

"I'm trying to find Colleen Clark, my mother. It's an *emergency*," I'd say. Or, "There's been an accident." I figured out the tricks that would get a response other than a hang up.

I'd hear someone shout for her, and if she wasn't there, a click and a dial tone would quickly follow.

I'd repeat the process until I heard my mother's voice on the line. "Why are you calling me?" she'd demand. "What's the emergency?"

"It's 12:30, Mom. I was worried."

"Just you go to bed, everything's fine," she'd say, knowing that I would remain at the front window, waiting for her car to pull up. When my mother finally arrived at the curb, I'd be like a parent, waiting the requisite three minutes for her to come in before flicking the porch lights on and off. If that didn't get her attention, I'd go outside and knock on the car windows—much to the surprise of her date. I'd puff out my chest a little to compensate for my soon-to-be-outgrown Batman pajamas. I had audacity for sure, but I also understood the unstated deal we'd made and I was holding her to it.

Though my dad disappeared when I was seven years old and all my siblings left me behind by the time I turned ten, I was not about to lose my mother. It was something I believed I could keep from happening through creativity and sheer will. I looked for and found ways to become valuable to her and needed, yet I also remained the little boy fighting for his mom. It was our bond.

Mom acted as if her romances were just a fun way to pass the time, but I knew she desperately wanted to be in love and she also wanted someone to take care of her. When she met Art, the traveling salesman, I sensed that this was something different. From the first moment he walked in the door, I liked him. I think it was a first.

After a couple of weeks, Mom started referring to Art as her boyfriend. Unfortunately, due to his job, he was only in town once every few weeks, and he didn't have a regular schedule. Mom would sit by the phone waiting for it to ring. When it finally did, she'd compose herself with a deep breath, then answer in her best carefree voice. If it was Art calling, she'd be happy for hours.

Whenever she got confirmation that Art was coming to town, Mom would skip around our little house and sing at the top of her lungs. She'd spend hours—literally—in front of the mirror, trying on dozens of different outfits. Art made her feel like a showgirl.

When the moment finally arrived and Art was at the door, Mom would nearly hyperventilate. I got excited when Art arrived, too. He usually brought something for me: sometimes a Hot Wheels car or a comic book. Then he'd take Mom's hand, bow low, and kiss her knuckles. They'd go to dinner. They'd go dancing. Mom would come home giggling, stumbling a little, and happy, as happy as I'd ever seen her. He seemed perfect.

Six months into their courtship, I asked Mom a question I'd been mulling for a while. "Is Art going to be my new dad?"

"Oh, my son," Mom said, shaking her head. "No, not right now anyway. Maybe someday."

I didn't understand. "Why someday? Why not now?"

"The truth is that Art already has a family. He has a wife and two kids in Spokane. But he's not happy with them. I think he wants to be with us. It will just take time, my son."

When Art stopped coming around, Mom didn't say a word. But when she went out on a date with someone else, I remember thinking: *Well, that must be the end of Art.* I missed him and wondered what would happen next, but there was a line I knew not to cross. Mom's realm of independence and good times was not to be breached.

Years later, Mom admitted to me that she loved Art and that she always thought of him as the best man she'd ever had in her life. She even called him her soul mate. That was the first time that I completely understood that Art was the love of her life and that their breakup had been a critical blow that had broken her heart for the last time.

I think for my mother, every guy that came after Art was nothing but a placeholder.

Visions of Aunt Joan

Over the two months following my birthday party, Edweena began calling more frequently with "reports" of my mother's forgetfulness. It was frustrating. Mom had missed an important appointment with her heart doctor, for example. She'd lost her keys. She'd mixed up the day of the week.

I found myself defending and denying that anything was wrong. "Mom's seventy-six years old," I'd argue, apparently willing to overlook Edweena's own credentials in behavioral matters, gained during a long career as a social worker. "You live that long and you've earned the right to forget things. Besides, she's been forgetful all her life. That's just the way she's wired."

I reminded my sister that this was a woman who could pull off a fabulous three-course meal with a fridge full of leftovers but had never been able to balance her checkbook or remember the names of the neighbors.

At regular medical checkups, Edweena had taken it upon herself to talk to Mom's doctor about these issues, but it wasn't adding up to more than the ordinary memory losses expected in an aging person.

Today's phone call, however, got my attention and left me thinking that maybe this was something more than Mom being her usual forgetful self. My sister is one of the strongest people I know, but the moment she came on the line, I detected the fatigue and worry in her voice. Something was different. Something was wrong.

47

She began by telling me that Mom had an "encounter" with our Aunt Joan, the sister who was not only Mom's closest in age but also her favorite. The two had much in common, having both married Americans and immigrated to the U.S., but Joan had died in 1972 at the age of forty-six.

"Last night I overheard Mom talking to Auntie Joan," Edweena announced. "Apparently Joan was furious with Mom for not visiting her and Mom got mad and told Joanie to shut up. Then Mom wandered right past me, outside, barefoot, wearing her pajamas. It was freezing cold."

Edweena had followed our mother and found her in the middle of the street, looking up at the stars. "I asked her what she was doing in the street without shoes," she continued. "Mom said that she just wanted to see the stars. Then she said it was nearly time for her to go visit Joan. I reminded her that Joan's been dead for years, but she just waved me away. Then she said she was hungry. 'Is it dinnertime yet? I'm starving.' I led her back inside and sat there while she ate a banana and then walked her to her room so she'd go to bed."

When Edweena finished her story, I didn't know what to say. My first instinct was to dismiss it as a gross exaggeration; something my family is prone to do. But I'd heard Edweena's strained, exhausted voice and I knew she wasn't stretching the truth. It had to have been real, too real.

Mom and Edweena have lived together in the same house in Post Falls, Idaho, just twenty-five miles east of Spokane, for over twenty-six years. Their relationship was more like that of sisters than mother and daughter. They did just about every-thing together. Sometime after her divorce, Edweena committed herself completely to Mom. She gave up on any dreams of hav-ing a romantic relationship or her own separate life. After this latest event, though, I wondered if even my resourceful social worker sister could manage Mom's care all by herself.

Mom wasn't just displaying unusual memory lapses and odd behavior. She had other health issues too. She had suffered several Transitory Ischemic Attacks (TIAs), episodes of neurologic dysfunction that are often referred to as mini-strokes and are not unusual among the elderly. She had also experienced other medical episodes. Edweena was forced to miss work because of all the minor and serious crises and was constantly on alert.

I didn't see what we could do. I lived six hours away. My other sister, Linda, was in California. Our brother, Larry, who did live nearby, had carved out a limited relationship with our family such that he was only available for holidays and occasional milestones. Since adolescence, he had determined that if he wanted to put his life and marriage first, he would need to pull away from Mom's charming and powerful grasp.

Edweena and I talked more, and she admitted that, most of the time, Mom was her normal self, just a little more out of it than usual. We'd been trying to keep Mom from drinking alcohol, the habit she'd picked up from her beau, Jack.

I had urged Edweena to push water on our mother, lots of it, in fact. "Staying hydrated is critical," I told her, recalling a lesson I'd learned from my earliest days of working with the elderly. "Dehydration can be a major cause of confusion."

Trying to be helpful, while delaying and denying my coming day of reckoning, I gave my sister some tips. "You could keep a glass of water around her and remind her to have a sip as often as possible, or maybe it would work to get her one of those 64-ounce water bottles that all the kids carry around." Secretly I wondered if she should be getting a weekly intravenous treatment of fluids to ensure she stayed hydrated.

(Studies have proven at the opposite end that too much hydration can be dangerous for the elderly. Older people have weaker heart muscles, dramatically reducing the ability to pump out excess fluid. If the heart can't pump the fluid out, then it builds up and can actually cause congestive heart failure. The best advice is to monitor that proper hydration levels are maintained.)

I bit my lip to keep from giving more advice.

There was a long pause between us and I heard my sister sigh in reply to my suggestions. I wanted to stress it again because it is so vitally important. Just a little water goes a long way in lubricating the connections of the brain. But I didn't say it. I didn't want to seem like I was preaching to Edweena.

"I just feel so alone, Dwayne," Edweena continued. "And I can't help her when I'm at work. I worry about her almost as if she was my child, and nothing I do really seems to help for very long. She's getting more and more dependent and anxious, not knowing when I'll get home, or overwhelmed trying to get through whatever she planned for the day. And I know she shouldn't be driving any more."

"What can I do?" I asked.

"I don't know," Edweena said. There was another long pause and then another heavy sigh. "I'm just so tired all the time."

"Maybe it's time to get a part-time caregiver to come to the house while you're working," I suggested. "I can cover it. It's what I can do to help."

Silence fell between us for a lengthy moment, but then Edweena conceded, "Yeah, maybe it's time for that. Mom would probably like the company."

Part 2.

Facing Change:
Cover Ups and Realities

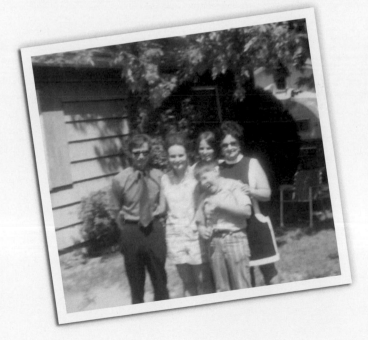

*Lewiston, Idaho 1969: Ron (brother-in-law), Linda,
Edweena, Colleen and Dwayne*

I love hearing my mother's stories of her etchze life in India. Fortunately to ten us, my grandmother lived with us for several years from the time I was about six years old, so Granny would help mom embellish her accounts of her teenage years in India.

^ You were either chasing after your father on studying fashion magazines for the latest trends in London or New York or Paris. Then you had to figure out her [...] while whatever [...] You certa[...] style [...] get ye[...] yes to [...] when I [...] your [...] always [...] until y[...] act ho[...] ink y[...] head [...] with [...] you [...] voice [...] and h[...]

India, 1935: Aunt Joan, Granddad and Colleen

SPREADING WINGS...AND A SPREADING SHADOW

It was destined to be a glorious day: The grand opening celebration of Aegis' second community. It had been twelve years since I'd first conceived the idea of my own assisted living company, and with the original facility thriving in Seattle, here we were, expanding already. Our second facility was located in Fremont, California, and we had plans to open six more in the coming year.

All my life, with my mother's support and inspiration, I'd dreamed of doing something that really mattered, something big. Finally, my hard work and well-orchestrated planning were paying off and my dreams were coming true. Rather than feeling overwhelmed, I felt relaxed and easy—something I hadn't really experienced before.

The day dawned perfect: 72 degrees, clear blue skies, and sunshine. The newly constructed building looked like something out of a storybook. The newly mown grass shone a luscious green, and the plants and flowers lining the front walk were in full bloom. Some 250 guests, including new residents and their families, attended.

We had booked a special, well-known guest: Jack LaLanne, an American health and exercise guru. At age eighty-five, Jack was still able to drop and crank out twenty pushups on command. As I said a few words at the official welcoming, I had to stop several times to catch my breath as I contemplated the fanfare surrounding this achievement. I can only compare it to the same sense of wonder I experienced when I saw my children take their first steps. We were spreading our wings, and I was filled with joy, gratitude, and hope.

After the announcements, and a few inspirational words by Jack, everyone ate lunch and toured from room to room. Some new residents began moving in. I met almost everyone in a dizzying melee of handshakes and hugs.

At one point, I tagged along with one of the tour groups that had stepped outside. The grounds behind the property featured a fantastic English garden. Looking over the gorgeous greenery, I thought of my mom and wished that Edweena had been able to drive her down, but it was one more burden she didn't need. Plus, I wasn't sure I was up for a possible crisis with my mom. But I wished that she could share all this with me. She would have a special appreciation for just how far I—and Aegis—had come.

On my drive to my hotel after a celebratory dinner, I was still buzzing from the energy of the day. The facts that I'd created this business from the germ of an idea, my plans had actually worked, and it was growing beyond me, like a living, breathing thing, all came together in my head and mixed with the warm nighttime air of California. I was experiencing the power of a great cliché: The American Dream. I felt completely relaxed behind the wheel as I cruised along. Nothing, I thought, could bring me down from this natural high. It was sublime.

Back in my room, I called Mom. As part of my regular routine, I always called her at least twice a week, as well as on special occasions, like this one. Of all the people in the world who could congratulate me on my success, she was the one I knew would touch me the most deeply.

Edweena picked up, her voice more tired than ever. I instantly felt an ache move through my gut. She had been crying.

"What is it, Dweena?" I asked. "What's the matter?"

"Mom fired the caregiver today," she started. "I finally felt like there'd be some help and here I had to come home from work early again."

"What happened? Why did she fire the caregiver? I thought she liked her."

"Mom was convinced that she stole from her," Edweena explained. "Her money. Her jewelry. Her car keys. Mom's been so paranoid lately. Even of me. She started to say that I'm conspiring against her with the caregiver to get her out of the house. I started crying and she stopped. A minute later, she didn't know why I was crying or what had happened. She was just totally confused, acting as if nothing was wrong." Edweena trailed off for a moment. Then I heard her blow her nose.

"We'll hire another caregiver," I assured her. "In fact, let's hire two. Whatever you need. You just tell me what you need."

"I'm sorry," Edweena said. "I'm just so tired."

Apparently, our mother had been up a lot at night lately, wandering. "She'll come into my room and crawl into bed with me and remind me that she's afraid of the dark," my sister explained. "Then she'll toss and turn and keep talking. She'll keep me up all night without a second thought. She just crawls into bed and talks and talks. She doesn't like to sleep alone because she doesn't always know where she is and she gets scared. Of course, she doesn't say it like that. I don't know if she's pretending or really believes she's okay. I honestly don't know if she's trying to cover things up, especially when she knows I'm mad and exhausted, or if she really doesn't realize how hard it is to be with her."

"Is she there? Can I talk to her?" I asked.

"Now's not a good time," Edweena said. "She's resting."

"Well, tell her I love her," I said. "Tomorrow we'll find some more help for you."

"How was your opening?" Edweena asked.

Given the sleepless nights and the emotional turmoil she was experiencing, Edweena still had the presence of mind to remember to ask about my special day. I couldn't believe it. "It was fine," I replied. I was going to provide details but stopped. Suddenly, it didn't seem very important. "You go try to get a little sleep," I told her. "We'll talk in the morning."

I hung up the phone and sat there on the edge of the hotel room bed, feeling empty. If my emotions were a penny, they'd just been flipped from heads to tails. As much as we'd tried not to believe it, Mom was increasingly exhibiting the classic symptoms of Alzheimer's disease.

I breathed in a few deep breaths and thought about Jack LaLanne doing pushups, one right after the other. Tomorrow, we'd find two new people to help care for Mom while Edweena was at work. I'd talk to Mom tomorrow on the phone and was sure that she—and everything else—would be just fine.

Maybe this is just a phase, I rationalized to myself. Even with that, though, I couldn't help but hear Mom's familiar admonishment in my head: "I'll come back to haunt you if you put me in an old folks' home." Of all the people who would make such an outrageous threat, I believed Mom to be the one person who would actually find a way to make it happen.

Despite my new status as head of a fast-growing regional chain of assisted living communities, I could not place my mother in institutionalized care. Edweena wasn't ready for it, and Mom would hate me for it.

Idaho 1970
Tasty Food

My mother would be home soon, and I was hungry. I could usually count on her to bring something home from her new employer, the Wrangler Steakhouse, to reheat on the stove; I would make curry and rice on the stove, the perfect mix for her contribution.

I rolled out of my beanbag chair where I was watching TV, turned up the volume so that I could hear every word of the "Gilligan's Island" rerun from the kitchen, and set to work.

Food was about the only thing that could take me away from my beloved television, my best friend. I was twelve years old, my pleasures still simple.

Tonight, I challenged myself: This would be the moment my mother finally admitted that I could cook "Tasty Food" to her highest standard, a fast, inexpensive culinary delight containing just the right amount of fat, salt, and grease to make it—to us— disastrously seductive.

I overheard the Professor explaining his latest invention to the Skipper and Gilligan even as I pulled a frying pan from the dishes stacked in the sink and scoured it with a soapy rag. After flicking the gas on and shaking the pan dry, I reached for the big can of reused bacon grease that was never far from the stove. I knew Mom's recipe for curry and rice by heart. She tossed ingredients in by sight and sense, never needing to measure. I suspected her intuitive cooking style was born less out of innate creativity than a need to improvise with what we had—but she never let it show.

I could smell that the bacon grease was just about warm enough to start cooking. First, the onions, then a couple of tablespoons of curry powder, plus an extra shake just to make sure it got Mom's attention, and then a little water once the onions had begun to brown and mingle with the curry powder. A good dose of ketchup would round out the thin stew that always tasted even better the second day. Next came the hard part, probably something that should have been on my mind before now: What should I throw in that could simmer into Tasty Food while I put the rice on to boil?

I was digging around in the refrigerator, discovering just how sparse the vegetable drawer's options were, when my mother came through the front door of our tiny house. "What's that god-awful smell in here? Time to take out the trash, my son!" I was sure she was kidding, but it wasn't always obvious.

"The best Indian curry you've ever had, Mom," I announced. Unfortunately, I hadn't found anything useful in the refrigerator to help my statement live up to its claim. "You bring anything to toss in, just in case?"

My mother seemed to fill the kitchen doorway: Her white cook's uniform amplified her sturdy frame and her elaborate hairdo must have added eight inches to her height. Her dress and shoes would have been reasonably clean when she had left for work in the morning, but a day of short-order cooking at the Wrangler had left her clothes spattered with beef blood, grease, gravy, and other ingredients inherent in the choices on a cheap-eats menu. Her bare arms bore the signature burn marks gained by anyone who ever made a living in front of a stove. Even at my tender age, it pained me to see those scars.

This was Mom's "work" persona: gritty, blue collar, and not afraid to get her kitchen uniform dirty. Mom's work and social lives were always in sharp contrast. Although she was fashion-conscious and wouldn't be caught dead if she wasn't dolled up for a night out, she had no qualms about showing up at my school in her stained cook's uniform during work hours.

While I respected my mother's work ethic, I was old enough by now to be embarrassed by her. Her uniform was a billboard, a neon sign advertising that she was stuck in a meaningless blue-collar job, blinking "low class" for all to see. I knew that my mother was better than that. We were better than that.

I recalled the time when she came straight from work to a parent-teacher conference. She had arrived during school hours, and I slid down in my seat to keep her from catching sight of and waving at me. Fortunately, the bell signaling the end of the school day rang without my teacher calling attention to the woman standing in the back of the class.

I had escaped potential mortification—or so I thought. As I sat and waited for the classroom to empty, leaving Mom and I alone with my teacher, I heard a classmate's voice call out. "Is that your mom back there, Dwayne?"

"Huh?" As if I wasn't interested in the topic. "Oh, uh, yeah. I guess so."

Tina looked at my mother in her bloodstained dress. "I didn't know she was a nurse."

"What?" Salvation. "Oh, that?" I shrugged, as if modesty pre-vented me from saying anything more about my mother's noble profession. The memory of it shames me today. She worked so hard for what little we had.

Now Mom waltzed into our kitchen, dropping her purse on the counter, eager to aid in my project. "Here you go." She handed me a brown, grease-stained paper bag. "Maybe that will save the mess you've got burning over there." I turned back to the stove and grabbed the handle of the smoking pan, dropping it instantly as I singed my bare fingers.

Mom rushed me to the sink and stuck my fingers under the cold running water as I started to whine. "That's nothing, it will just be a blister to remind you for a few days to be more careful. The mark of a real cook, my son."

"Yes, my mother." I said, the "my mother" in my response dripping with unconcealed sarcasm, as it almost always did whenever she used the stilted phrase "my son" in conversation. She didn't respond. In fact, my mother never rose to my implied taunt, never justified the formality of her words, and never used the phrase in a context that implied any particular emotion, whether good or bad. I was her son, and it was her right to declare me so.

My mother was ready to eat. "Are you going to finish what you started, or do I have to turn this into something worth eating myself?"

She would often bring home scraps and leftovers from the kitchen, having carefully cut around partially eaten steak or pork chops that customers had not finished, sometimes with teeth marks still visible. Mom would tell her coworkers that she was making a doggie bag, but of course, these meager treats were for our consumption. This habit may have taken the "one man's trash is another man's treasure" philosophy a bit too far, but she wasn't going to let perfectly good food go to waste while we had so little at home. Tonight was no exception. I picked up the bag from the counter where it had fallen and peeked inside.

"Cool! Meatballs!"

"They were the buffet special," Mom explained. "Not as popular today as usual, so they weren't going anywhere."

I broke the leftover meatballs up and dropped them into the pan to brown. Curry, meatballs, and rice. It would be classified as a poor man's food in Lewiston, Idaho, but it was Tasty Food to me—even if my mother still didn't agree.

October 2000
"Don't Eat the Pie"

Looking back now, what should have been a relatively normal autumn week for my feisty, enthusiastic seventy-seven-year-old mother instead provided the first hints that the journey through her golden years would not be smooth. Rather, it would be fraught with unexpected bumps, snags, turnarounds, and mis-direction, and we, her family, soon realized that there was no map available that could help us navigate the way.

The trouble started after Mom went to Jack's on one of her regular visits. Every few weeks, she somehow managed to get Edweena to make the five-hour drive to his house north of Seattle to drop her off and then, a few days later, make the same round-trip drive to bring her home.

This most recent visit had not provided the good times Mom always anticipated. Instead, according to Jack, Mom sud-denly started feeling dizzy and nauseous and then got worse and worse until she felt so bad that she was lying on the floor, barely conscious. Jack called a cab and rushed her to the Everett hospital, where she was admitted. An emergency room physi-cian called for a battery of tests and determined that she had suffered a Transient Ischemic Attack (TIA), or a minor stroke, the first of what would turn out to be many for my mother. For three days she remained in the hospital for observation. When no further complications arose, they released her.

Edweena drove down to help with her discharge from the hospi-tal and the trip home. Relieved that Mom was given a clean bill of health, Edweena, Mom and I met for breakfast at the Brown Bag, a small diner in Redmond.

The parking lot proved unusually busy, and in the melee of cars trying to angle into spaces, Edweena nudged the car ahead of her. The driver emerged, spitting angry and screaming curses and threats at my sister, who had stepped out to inspect for any damage. Before I could do anything, Mom jumped out herself and stood between them, a mother bear protecting her cub.

"Hey asshole!" she yelled. "What kind of man are you, yelling at a lady? You're a coward!"

The man took a step back, shocked by this furious, tiny, nearly eighty-year-old woman in his face. She jabbed a finger into his chest before I could get to her and lead her away. Bewildered, the man quickly calmed down, conceded that there was no damage to his car, and gave Edweena the parking spot.

We went in and sat down. The restaurant was very busy and waiters buzzed around the room. Mom's blood was still boiling, even after we found our seats and started sipping water. I tried to change the topic, suggesting that we head over to the mall for some shopping after lunch, but even that didn't help. Mom glared at the rude guy who'd yelled at Edweena. He was sitting across the room, engrossed in a menu. I rubbed Mom's hand and encouraged her to relax, but then her physical demeanor took a sudden, terrifying turn. She announced that she might faint and, as I looked at her, the color drained from her face.

Edweena and I stood up at the same time. Mom's eyes fluttered and she slowly slumped over, into my arms. I lowered her to the carpet, pocked with old coffee stains and strewn with breadcrumbs. I cradled her head as Edweena ran for help. After admonishing my mother to wake up, I tried gently slapping her cheek, but when she didn't respond, I felt my stomach sink like an elevator.

Two police officers, in line to pay their bill, saw what was happening and raced over. They dropped to my side and I stepped back, assuming that they would begin CPR. I was in shock now. My vision appeared gauzy and my body felt heavy, as if I were wading through mud. One officer radioed for help while the other firmly pressed two fingers against Mom's neck.

"No pulse," he announced, looking up at his partner.

The partner pursed his lips and bowed his head. They traded glances and shrugged their shoulders. The one who'd taken Mom's pulse looked at me with resignation and sorrow written on his face. It was only then that I realized they weren't going to do anything more. To them, she was just an old woman who had died while they were on their lunch break. End of story.

Think, think, think! I ordered myself as I tried to focus and figure out what to do. Twenty years prior, I had been certified as a CPR instructor. Though I'd never used the life-saving procedure in a real-life situation, my instincts, coupled with a white-hot flame of adrenaline, took over.

I grabbed the officer who had taken Mom's pulse and shoved him aside, sending him crashing into a nearby table. His partner, still kneeling at my side, didn't make any move to stop me. Hovering over my mother, I put my ear to her mouth and nose to listen and feel for breath. Nothing. I scooped out her dentures, feeling the crumbs of bread she hadn't swallowed. Maybe I should have left them in. They might make a better breathing seal. No. Too late for that. I'd already lost precious time.

"Starting CPR," I said to no one in particular. I tilted her head back and blew three breaths into her lungs. Nothing. I looked at her lips. They were turning blue. I'd kissed her a thousand times before on the cheek and here I was putting my mouth over hers for a final, desperate farewell.

No! You're not going to die on me, Mom. Not here.
Not like this.

I gasped for air. Thoughts raced through my mind as I unbuttoned the top buttons of Mom's blouse and parted the fabric to reveal her skin. I put one hand over the other and began manual compressions. I counted out loud.

"One." *If I push too hard, I'll rupture her sternum.*

"Two." *I can't be the one doing this.*

"Three." *I want to go into the corner and curl into a ball.*

"Four." *My mother is dying. She may already be dead.*

I pinched her nose and prepared to give her a couple more puffs of air. I lowered my mouth to hers. Then without warning, her eyes popped open. Oh, what relief as she gripped my hand, an absolutely pure rush of warmth that went straight to my heart and filled me up.

Only now, as I looked up did I see that everyone in the restaurant was watching the drama unfold. For a moment, the audience sat in absolute silence. Then Mom coughed, just once. She looked around and saw all eyes on her.

"Don't eat the pie," she quipped, not missing a beat.

The diner erupted with laughter and applause. I held it together as best I could and told Mom that she'd just fainted, but that she was fine now. No big deal. Edweena gave me her coat and I put it under Mom's head. Mom took my hand and winked at me, and I chuckled. It took all my strength to keep from breaking down. The policemen waited with us. We kept saying how lucky it was that they were there even though they hadn't done anything substantive. We needed to say something to ease the tension and calm our nerves.

A few minutes later, the paramedics arrived. They conducted a quick examination of Mom before putting her on a gurney. She didn't appreciate the fuss, but she took a shine to the driver. As she was loaded into the ambulance, Mom touched his arm and jokingly suggested, "Why don't you ride in back with me?"

Edweena and I followed the ambulance to the hospital in our own cars. My head was swimming with a rush of adrenaline I'd never felt before. Outside my window, life went on. A group of kids chased each other down the street. Several people stepped off a bus. A couple kissed outside a coffee shop. I could feel my own pulse pounding in my ears as emotions pinballed around my gut and chest. I felt grateful and overjoyed yet also afraid and despondent. I thought about my own children. I thought about life and the thin string of hope we all live by.

At the hospital, the doctors determined that Mom's heart was having trouble maintaining its natural rhythm due to a malfunction in the intrinsic electrical conduction system. Essentially, this meant that she wasn't getting the energy she needed to power her heart muscle.

They immediately wheeled her into surgery and implanted a pacemaker. Afterward, when she had been stabilized, we were allowed to see her. Edweena and I both stopped at the threshold to take in the scene. My mother lay motionless in a hospital bed as half a dozen tubes ran from her body back to a bank of machines that included heart monitors, IV fluids, and oxygen.

As we approached the bed, her eyes fluttered open. Very slowly, she reached for my hand as I neared her bed. I'd promised myself I'd be strong for her, but with the shock of seeing the tubes and hearing the chirps of her life-support equipment all around me, I had difficulty staying cool.

Then her hand touched mine. "The doctors say you saved my life," she informed me. "See that? I knew I brought you up right. Thank you, my son."

I told my mother how much I loved her. "It's okay, my son," she said. "I'm going to be just fine."

INDIA 1938
DADDY'S GIRL

Mom had always been a survivor, an identity that she could trace back to those tenuous first moments of life. It was at St. Mary's Parochial School, however, that she really honed her skills. The nuns there could be harsh, and she frequently told me about how she dreamed of being rescued from there. She never learned to live harmoniously with the holy sisters, who in that time and place were obliged to try to tame her and may have even gotten some kind of perverse pleasure from their efforts.

Most of Mom's stories ended with a description of the punishment she received, but somehow she managed to stay at St. Mary's for nearly ten years. It just didn't seem to be within her capacity to follow the nuns' rules, reasonable or not. I have often wondered how different—for better or worse—Mom's life might have been if she'd been more receptive to the lessons they tried to teach her.

"At night I'd curl up in my bunk and pull Father's handkerchief out from under my pillow." She would demonstrate holding the cloth up to her face and breathe in deeply, lost in the memory. "It never seemed to lose his smell, the mix of cherry-leaf tobacco and aftershave. It gave me something to look forward to, the day each semester when he would arrive on the train and take me away from that horrible place."

And so, at the end of each semester, her dreams *would* come true, at least for a few weeks. Back at home, Mom would tag along with her father, finding excuses to be around him. Mom's time working in her father's office offered a stark contrast to her life at the convent school. Of course, that was partly because, at the office, Mom got her orders from someone that she wanted desperately to please. And without doubt, my grandfather indulged her longings and impulses. "I don't remember how much he paid me to do the little jobs he assigned, but I needed every penny of it to supplement what I could squeeze out of Mother for the latest fashions," she told me.

I never tired of hearing my mother recite stories of her exotic life in India. Fortunately, my grandmother lived with us for several years from the time I was about six years old, so Granny would help Mom embellish the accounts of her teenage years in India.

"You were either chasing after your father or studying fashion magazines for the latest trends in London or New York or Paris," I recall Granny telling my mother. "Then you had to figure out how to make it work with whatever was at hand in India. You certainly had your own style and you managed to get your father to say yes to all of your whims. When I tried to say no to your latest request, I would always tell you, 'Just you wait until your father comes home,' but he would laugh and give into you. It was nice that you had such a happy relationship with your father."

Granny's voice caught at the memory. "He enjoyed your admiration—and he deserved it!"

When she was fifteen, Mom graduated from St. Mary's and took a job as a nanny for a British doctor, which, it turned out, was a perfect role for her. The work was fun and relatively easy. Moreover, she was close to home and, with her job, was able to maintain the independence she'd developed while away at school.

Granny and Mom loved to talk about my grandfather, but they rarely spoke about his death. It was a singular trauma for each of them. Apparently, my grandfather had ignored his doctor's warning that even a mild case of malaria required bedrest and care. Instead of staying at home to recuperate, he continued to go to work, having declared himself "fit as a fiddle."

"It was such an unfair death," Granny declared on one of the few times they did discuss the details. "His stubbornness led the doctors to prescribe a double dose of quinine to help him resist the disease while working long days at the office. It almost seemed funny when the chronic hiccups first started, but then they just kept on, day after day."

Granny continued in a near whisper. "After a while, he could barely breathe. His stomach muscles were cramping so badly that he couldn't stand. After the fourth day, he collapsed and we took him to the hospital. There didn't seem to be anything anyone could do, other than wait and hope they would subside on their own."

Mom had put her arm around Granny. "You certainly did everything you could. I remember you were by his bedside day and night."

"But you and your sister Joan were there almost as much as I was," remembered Granny. "Except on that last day. You'd gone home for a few hours to clean up and eat. It was his gift to you, you know. He spared you the final moments," she sighed.

Mom spoke up with force. "I'll never forgive myself for not being there with him—and with you."

Apparently, my mother arrived back at the hospital at the very moment they were taking her father to the morgue. One of the attendants lazily kicked the gurney down the hall, and Mom became furious. She ran to the attendant, took him by the lapel, and shook him. "Hey you!" she screamed through a veil of tears. "That's my father. Do you hear me? My father! You treat him with respect!"

The family was devastated by my grandfather's sudden and strange death. I always thought it precipitated my mother's lifelong fear of dying—a dread rivaled only by her fear of being alone. At that point in the story, I remember vividly my mother turning away and staring off into the distance. "Everything changed after that. It all seemed to become so much harder," she said softly.

YARD SALE

Mom was always feisty. She never shied away from saying or doing exactly what she wanted. I suppose it was because she didn't have many social "filters" and she didn't seem to need anyone's approval. "I don't give a rat's ass what they think!" she would declare, citing what was to be one of her signature sayings. If anyone dare shoot a comment back in her direction, she'd be nonplussed: "Well, that rolls off me like water on a duck's ass," she'd quip.

Now, though, there seemed to be something more than feistiness at work; there was an unpredictable edge that lurked just beneath the surface. Was it Jack's continued influence? Was it the drinking? Was it her "true" nature finally coming to full flower? Edweena was bearing the brunt of Mom's unpredictably, neediness, and confusion. Still, they remained inseparable except for Mom's visits with Jack and continued to enjoy time together as "bingo queens" and garage sale aficionados.

Personally, I have no interest in garage sales. Who wants to spend all week setting one up and then sit around all day waiting for the opportunity to dicker over the cost of a 15 year-old can opener? Nonetheless, I needed to do a big house cleaning to get rid of years of accumulated clutter, and when I mentioned it to Edweena, I wasn't surprised that she grabbed the ball and ran with it. It seemed like the kind of fun project that would bring out the best in my mom and would get them both away from their own house, which was taking on a pall of stress and anxiety.

They immediately started planning, and it took just minutes for me to realize that the whole thing was now out of my hands. I loved to see them like this: a modern-day Lucy and Ethel obsessing over a crazy new project. After reminding them to call if they needed anything and assuring them that any profits were theirs to keep, I excused myself.

The day before the sale, Edweena and my mom got down to business. It turned out that I couldn't quite escape the madness. "What do you think we should ask for this fireplace screen, Dwayne?" Edweena asked me, just as I made my way back into the house.

"I dunno. Ten dollars?" I was trying to remember where it had come from. I looked over the stacked piles of stuff waiting to be claimed by new owners or donated to Goodwill and realized I couldn't really remember where any of it had come from, much less the original cost or current value.

"Are you crazy?" my mother shot back at me. "That's solid brass. I bet it's an antique. Edweena, I think we should label it as $49.99 and be willing to take $35."

"I agree," Edweena had said, pulling out a green label from a packet of assorted colors. "Green's for furnishings," she explained to me. Mom was already pouring through the artwork, with a sheet of red labels in hand. "Edweena, how do you want to handle the display of these pictures?" Mom had asked and then, turning to me, said, "I think we're fine here, son." Clearly, I had been dismissed.

The day of the sale was picture perfect. The skies sparkled blue, but it was warm, not hot. I surveyed the driveway and wasn't at all surprised to see the discarded troves laid out like lost treasures. Just like Edweena, I thought. I merely mentioned that I had some stuff to unload and here we were with a professional-caliber yard sale, perfectly envisioned, and meticulously arranged.

74

Mom and Jack didn't arrive until early afternoon, having called earlier to let us know they were stopping for lunch, thus handily avoiding the actual work of selling stuff. By the time they arrived at the house, most of the items were gone and I was trying to convince Edweena to close up early so I could take her out for a nice meal.

When I saw my mother get out of the car, I noticed right away that something was a little off. She was overly animated and hyped up as she picked through the remains of the sale. I reminded myself that she often acted like a teenager around Jack, swept away by his charms.

Mom moved through the unsold items and quickly noticed an old exercise bike near the fringe of the grass—it was just too out-of-date to be of much use to today's fitness buffs. She suddenly climbed aboard and started pedaling, looking up and waving at us. She began shouting, "Hey, look at me! Check it out! I'm in the best shape of my life!"

Jack smirked and waved back at her absently and went back to picking through a box filled mostly with old golf balls.

As Mom sped up her peddling, Edweena and I exchanged amused glances. We were both happy to see her having fun and relieved since, in months past, she'd been acting more and more anxious and moody. But then she began pedaling faster.

"Hey! Look at me go!" she shouted, louder than before. We all stared at her, including the few customers who were still poking around, not sure of what to make of the scene. There was no way she could keep up her frantic pace. I started toward her, but it was too late. In an instant, the pedals came out from under her feet and flipped her flat on her back onto the grass.

I knelt beside her as she tried to get up. "Just stay put for a second, Mom," I said, putting a gentle hand on her shoulder.

"Oh bloody hell!" she said, embarrassed. "I'm fine. I'm fine. I can't believe I let that thing get the better of me."

"Don't worry," I said. "Are you hurt?"

"I'm fine," she said and tried to get up.

I kept my hand on her shoulder and, as I leaned closer, I noticed three distinct and alarming realities: I could detect the unmistakable scent of alcohol, dense on her breath. There was a clump of what looked like mud on her shoe and seemed out of place. Overpowering the moment was a distinctive and powerful smell: feces. In one horrible instant, I realized that it wasn't mud on my mom's shoe. I think Mom realized what happened too because she wouldn't meet my eyes and tried again to push my hand away as I helped her to her feet. Edweena was standing over us now.

"Oh, Mom," Edweena said. "What's happened here?"

"Nothing," Mom said. "What do you mean? Just let me up on the bike again. I'll show it who's boss."

On her feet, my mother teetered for a moment. Edweena and I both helped steady her. The stench overwhelmed my senses, and I reflexively stepped back, suddenly feeling out of my own body, sapped of strength. Thank God my sister didn't miss a beat.

"C'mon, Mom," Edweena said. "Let's go inside and get you cleaned up."

"Oh," my mom said, absently. "I must have stepped in something."

"No problem, Mom," Edweena said, like nothing had happened as she led her inside.

Edweena caught my eye, but she gave nothing away.

My mother let Edweena lead her into the house. Jack was standing off to one side, unconcerned. He shrugged before picking up one of the old golf clubs still for sale and taking a long, slow-motion practice swing. "This is all his fault," I reasoned to myself.

I was possessed by the desire to snatch the club from his hands and beat him with it. I need to get out of here, I thought. I left a neighbor in charge and took off down the street.

"That son of a bitch is killing my mom," I raged to myself, moving quickly down the sidewalk to put as much distance as possible between him and me. He's ruining her, turning her into an alcoholic. It seemed the only two things Edweena, Linda, and I talked about in our phone calls these days was how to get Mom to quit drinking—and how to get her to quit Jack. Because when she isn't drinking, when she isn't with him, she's fine. But then come these crazy, sad, humiliating episodes and we can always find Jack or an empty, hidden bottle not far away.

But a nagging fear kept pushing into my thoughts. What if the problem wasn't just the drinking? I've worked around people with dementia for most of my adult life and the behavior my mother was exhibiting seemed uncomfortably familiar. In fact, alcohol abuse and dementia can feed off each other. Excessive drinking can certainly bring on dementia and can exacerbate fuzzy thinking and confusion. On the other hand, some people who begin to notice their memories failing begin to rely on alcohol to help them feel a sense of control. And anyone who has a couple of drinks to help their memory is likely to take a third drink and a fourth. Suddenly, they're drunk and deluded, leaving them in worse shape than ever. Like my mom, I thought.

But I flipped the conundrum over one more time. No one knows if a person with dementia will think any more clearly without the drinking, and what value is there in soberness—or even healthy eating—at a certain stage of life? Would it really make a difference? All the coulds and shoulds I've known as a professional were thrown out the window when I began to face the very same issues in my own life with my own mom.

Eventually I stopped walking, closed my eyes, and tilted my head back to feel the fading sun on my face. *I have to keep it together,* I thought. Speculating and worrying isn't going to make this better. We need to get Mom to stop drinking.

I walked back to the house, and when I got there, Mom and Edweena were still inside. Jack was trying out another golf club, an old pitching wedge I never used.

"How much you asking for this?" he said.

"You want it, just take it," I said sharply.

As I watched him smile, I felt dizzy from all the emotions swirling inside of me. I was furious. And afraid. And maybe most of all, guilty. I felt like I was letting my mom down but I didn't know what to do.

A few minutes later, she emerged from the house alone. She walked right past me, head down, without saying a word.

"Hey, Mom," I said. "You okay?"

"I'm fine, my son," she said quietly. "It'll take more than a little spill to put me out of action."

Jack showed her the golf club I'd given him and they talked about where they wanted to go for dinner. A woman approached and asked if I'd take $15 for the bike. My mother overheard this and looked back over her shoulder.

"Oh yeah," she piped in, always the tough negotiator. "It's a bargain at that price."

I realized I couldn't blame Jack alone. What I was really feeling was anger at myself for not doing more for my mom *and* for

Edweena. I hadn't let myself see the burden she'd been carrying. When I went to bed that night, I couldn't sleep. I couldn't stop replaying the terrible moment of Mom falling off the bike and what came after. My mother was becoming a stranger to me.

Idaho 1970
A Gift for Mom

Mom always had big dreams for me and I always knew she meant for me to be a big success—big being defined as money, a "you've made it" title, and social status. I suppose she hoped to reap some vicarious benefits for herself too. It wasn't clear that I would ever fulfill her "big shot" dreams, but I would have an early start trying.

When I turned eleven, I got my first real job. Our house was six blocks from the Arctic Circle, the local drive-in diner where I loved to tag along with my sister and hang out after school with my friends. We would pedal our banana-seat Stingrays over and watch the high school kids tear the place up. Some days there were fistfights, but more often, there were food-fights. It could start with a single French fry, but within moments, the air would be swarming with half-eaten burgers, milkshakes, and little paper cups full of ketchup. By the time the kids rumbled out of the lot in a convoy of cruisers, the fast-food mess was everywhere, even on the windows and walls.

I didn't see a disgusting mess, though. I saw entrepreneurial opportunity. After the parking lot cleared each day, I would watch the manager, Billy, who must have weighed 350 pounds, as he picked up the trash, cursing under his breath the entire time. It was a struggle for him with all the bending down. Clearly, he hated this aspect of his work. So when I approached him and proposed that he pay me to pick up the trash after school, he jumped at the chance. I earned two dollars per day, no matter how long it took me, and a big bonus—all the French fries I could eat.

Every day after school, I gathered up my slop bucket, some rags, a scrub brush, and a broom and got to work. It wasn't easy. The pigeons dive-bombed me for stealing their dinner and the high school kids treated me like I was their personal butler. If I didn't respond to their requests for a napkin or a cup of water, they'd sling tartar sauce at the wall, knowing I'd have to wash it off. But I didn't care. I was making money. Now I just had to figure out what to spend it on.

A week or two after I started working at the Arctic Circle, I went to the Mini-Mart and bought candy and comic books and brought them home to show off my earned treasure. No one showed much interest, and I ended up eating up too much candy and making myself ill. The comics and baseball cards gave me some enjoyment, but I wasn't a collector, and after a while, spending my money on these things seemed frivolous. I decided to focus on something more substantial.

That something came to me one day after my shift as I was walking around downtown. In front of me was a picture window of a dress shop with a pair of smartly dressed mannequins posed in mid-stride. The backdrop was a Paris cityscape, complete with the Eiffel Tower. It struck me as elegant.

"Of course," I said to myself. "Something for Mom."

Making her happy was like candy to me. It sounds corny now, but it was true then. I just loved to see Mom happy. And there, in front of me, was—to my mind—an obvious way to make my mother smile. For days, if not years.

Clothes had long held a special magic for Mom. She could spend hours trying on clothes in front of the mirror. It was her way of relaxing and letting go. Buying her some new clothes seemed the perfect way to spend my newfound wealth.

I took a last look at the strutting mannequins and smiled as I imagined Mom right up there with them, cutting through the streets of Paris in a suit I had purchased for her.

The young saleswoman approached me slowly as I looked through the racks of women's clothes. "Are you lost, son?" she asked, hands folded over her chest.

"No," I said. "I'm shopping."

"Oh, I see," she said, smugly. There was a note of arrogance and aggravation in her voice. She seemed to be assessing me carefully and wondering how I could possibly afford to buy anything.

"For my mom . . . for a gift," I explained.

The woman's tone changed immediately and gave way to a much more helpful demeanor. Before I could say another word, she went to her co-worker and explained my situation. They both cooed over me, thinking it adorable, and they brought out scarves and several pairs of gloves. I knew my mom would love all the things they showed me, but I was thinking bigger. She had been in this store many times, spending hours trying on items that were too expensive and always leaving empty-handed.

"No thanks," I said. "I'd like to buy her a suit."

Surprised, they looked at each other, then back at me. One of them finally asked, "A suit?"

"Actually, I'd like to make it two," I said. "Two suits, please. My mom's a perfect size ten." And by that time, I'd found them. I pointed at the two best-looking suits in the shop. One was on a mannequin. It was navy, trimmed in white, with gaps in the sleeves and big white buttons. Navy was formal and stately, I thought. The second suit hung from a display along the far wall. It was a party-suit, colored two shades of peach and cut just above the knee.

"And how are you going to afford those?" the younger sales-woman asked suspiciously.

"I have money," I stated and reached into my front jeans pocket. Billy paid me in cash, always in one-dollar bills, and I had saved for at least three weeks before I came into the shop. The result-ing wad of bills was so big that I once I wrapped my fingers around it I couldn't get my hand out of my pocket. The shop ladies giggled as I tugged and struggled to pull my hand free. I'm sure it was all very funny, but I was trying to conduct busi-ness and desperate to be taken seriously. I braced myself and gave a mighty pull. Suddenly, dollar bills burst out and floated to the ground and I squatted immediately to gather them up. The ladies immediately stopped laughing and locked onto my eleven-year-old fist clutching a fortune in dollar bills. We talked about a layaway plan. I think I became their favorite customer.

Every Saturday morning, I would get up and ride my bike to the store to make my payment on those suits, always with a hefty stack of dollar bills. If I wasn't going to make it that week, or if I had something else I had to do, I would call the shop ladies, Phyl-lis and Edith, to let them know I'd be there the following week. Over the several months it took me to buy the suits, those women became like aunts to me. I looked forward to seeing them and to our chats about my schoolwork and friends and their families. One week when I came in, they asked me to come to the back room. They had something new to talk about with me.

"You're a good boy," Phyllis began. "Your mom is very lucky to have a son like you."

"Yes, you're a good son," Edith agreed. "We've decided you don't have to make your last three payments. We're waiving them. So you can take the suits home today. You're done now. And we're very proud of you."

Walking out of the boutique with the wrapped boxes under my

arm was the proudest moment of my young life. My mother's birthday was still a few months away so I had to hide the boxes. I remember moving them from room to room, always thinking that the previous hiding place wasn't quite good enough.

When her actual birthday finally arrived and she opened the first box with the navy suit, Mom was confused. She held it up and considered it, front and back. She looked at me and frowned. How could her young son afford to buy such an expensive gift?

"It's brand new," she stated.

"I saved up from my trash job," I said.

"You saved to buy this for me? A dollar at a time?"

"Yep."

"Oh, my son." She started to cry. "Oh, my son. It's the best gift anyone has ever given me. I just can't believe it."

That's when I handed her the second box.

Later, I watched her try the suits on for the first time. She twirled and posed and, occasionally, looked back over her shoulder and blew me a kiss.

I remember her saying one of her trademark lines: "Hubba hubba, bling bling, Baby you've got everything." I laughed. Then she added, "People tell me I look like Elizabeth Taylor— only prettier!" I loved seeing her so happy.

Over the years, she wore her suits to many occasions, and I always felt a wave of pride wash over me when I saw her come out of her room dressed in either one. She'd always make a show of them in front of me, sashaying by me as if she were on a catwalk in Paris. She'd stop and turn sharply, the way runway models do, and then march by me in the opposite direction, always turning and looking at me and saying something like "fabulous" or "extraordinary."

I think she genuinely liked the suits, but I can't say for certain. Maybe she did. Or maybe they became a symbol to her, an emblem of what is possible if your faith is greater than your fear.

Or maybe she wore the suits for me. Just to tell me she loved me. Any of those reasons was fine with me.

SPRING 2002
QUEEN FOR A DAY

I had a plan to help Edweena. It was also a plan, I suppose, to take away some of my guilt and have more quality time with my mother. My wife, Terese, and I would take Mom for a whole two weeks while Edweena and our sister, Linda, took a fabulous trip to Europe.

I was so excited that Edweena had the energy to even imagine such a grand adventure. She'd been carrying an almost unbearable load—years of being at Mom's beck and call, doing all the shopping, arranging, and managing, as well as enduring endless miles of chauffeuring since Mom had stopped driving. The caretaking had gone from "helping" to something much more. Mom wasn't just old: She seemed to be declining rapidly. Love and duty had compelled Edweena to stretch far beyond her limits. The least I could do was take Mom while Dweena received a long-overdue respite.

So while Edweena and Linda were in Europe, Mom stayed with us. I had actually been looking forward to her visit, thankful to be able to spend some uninterrupted time together. Not since my children were young had we spent more than a night or two together. I imagined taking time off work and enjoying a series of "good days" with her. Despite my professional experience, I had no idea how much work it would be to care for Mom.

Terese and I dropped Edweena off at the airport before we brought Mom to our house and got her situated in the guest room. Edweena had given me extensive instructions on the state

87

of Mom's health, her many medications, including the one for anti-anxiety, and how much to give her and when; and what to do if she started wandering around the house.

Mom looked very frail, and Terese, a registered nurse, noticed that she was quite a bit thinner. To our relief, though, she seemed quite happy to be at our house. She sat in the kitchen chatting as we prepared dinner and when we sat down for a fine meal of Mom's favorites, she ate well. However, Edweena quickly came up in conversation, along with some previously undetected anxiety. Mom couldn't understand why Edweena had to go away without her. She felt left behind.

"But Mom," I explained, "we wanted you to ourselves. We want to spoil you a little."

That made her smile and the conversation picked up as we listed some of the fun things we could do this week, like shopping, which perked her right up. After dinner, we relaxed and watched "America's Most Wanted," Mom's favorite show, my mother in the leather reclining chair and Terese curled up next to me, reading a book. I felt like a kid again, gathered around the television with my family. All we were missing was Herman the wiener dog.

When Mom started looking sleepy, I gave her a hug and walked her up to her room.

"Good night, my son," she smiled warmly up at me. "Sweet dreams!"

She is so much like her old self, I thought, *and she isn't drinking.* Such a relief. I crawled into bed, happily imagining that we could possibly fatten her up a little during her stay. But then, as I started drifting off to sleep, random, anxious thoughts began to take over: *I wonder if Mom is alright in her room? What if I can't hear her and she's awake and doesn't know where she is?*

Finally I got out of bed and walked quietly down the hall to her room, listening outside her door to make sure she was asleep. I couldn't hear anything. She might have gotten up and started wandering around the house. I carefully opened the door, trying not to make a sound, and once I was in her room I could hear the gentle, regular sounds of her breathing. Relieved, I laughed quietly at myself and walked back to bed. An hour and a half later, I was awake again and couldn't do anything about it until I'd crept one more time into my mother's room and listened to her breathing. I repeated the ritual a couple more times that night and woke exhausted, thanks to my heightened awareness, exactly what I had experienced whenever there was a new baby in the house, that piercing sense of the fragility of life.

Fortunately, my mother woke up in a great mood. After we finished a big breakfast, I said, "Mom, let's go grocery shopping and get some of your favorite foods in the house."

"Good idea," Terese agreed. "We can use some milk, too."

We climbed into the car and headed to a gourmet shop nearby, where the displays in the shop looked more like abstract art than groceries.

I glanced at my mom, who looked tired but alert, like a kid in a candy store. "You know what I think, Mom? I think it's time we splurge. Let's get every dessert you've ever wanted. Everything you ever thought you wanted to taste—let's do it!"

She started to protest, but a mischievous smile was creeping over her face. I pulled a cart over and asked, "Which way first?"

She thought for a moment and said, "Remember the great key lime pie I used to make? I'd add strawberries to it and put it in the freezer and you'd eat the whole thing! I wonder if they have key lime pie?"

We went to the dessert section and there it was, along with a deep-dish apple pie and a Bavarian cream. I asked for one of each.

"Dwayne, we can't do that!" my mom exclaimed.

"Sure we can," I grinned. "No guilt or budgets today, Mom!" I had decided this would be a day for Tasty Food, just like old times.

"Oh, look at those!" my mom said, peering at an assortment of exquisite pastries, her eyes as wide as a little girl's.

"Let's get them all!" I cried. She looked at me like I was crazy, so I just shrugged and smiled. "Okay, you pick the best ones."

"But I'm going to get so big you'll have to roll me home!" she protested, even as she chose a lemon tart, a raspberry mousse, an orange crème bombe, and dark chocolate-covered strawberries.

We headed through the rest of the aisles, where my mom picked up and dropped barbecue chips, a wedge of Brie cheese, and a chunk of English cheddar into our cart.

When we got home, she took an inventory—the way she always did with important purchases—relishing each item as much as she did when she decided to buy it. We stashed everything in the cupboards and refrigerator before we had to explain ourselves to Terese.

"Ready to go real shopping now, Mom?" I asked. "We could head over to Bellevue." My mother reached for her purse and grinned. "I was born ready," she stated. As I drove into the parking garage of Bellevue Square, a nearby luxury shopping mall, I asked, "How does Nordstrom sound?"

"Just fine, son," she said.

As we entered the store, my mom took my hand and began to hum "Pennies from Heaven," which the pianist was playing on the floor above, and we strolled along together as if it was a day in the park. In the cosmetics section, we passed through fragrances hanging in the air like fruit from a tree. Eventually a brightly colored arrangement of designer silk scarves caught my mom's eye, and the store's personal stylist laid out a selection for her on the glass counter. My mother leafed through them carefully, and then smiled at the saleswoman, thanked her, and turned to go. "Do you like that one, Mom?" I pointed to one she had picked up several times.

"It's lovely, son, but we can't afford that," she whispered, smiling at the stylist and turning once again to go.

"Sure we can, Mom," I said, pulling out my wallet. My mother beamed as the saleswoman expertly wrapped the scarf in tissue and handed her the bag.

"Where to next?" I asked.

We set off through the store as if we were on a mission, exploring every department, stopping at each interesting display. In one of the designer departments, my mother tried on a beautiful teal suit. She hesitated as she came out from the dressing room; I think the hushed and almost empty department intimidated her.

"You look lovely," said our personal stylist, who had selected the suit for my mother.

Reassured, Mom looked at herself in the mirror and couldn't help but strike her signature model pose, thoroughly pleased with herself, as if she were ready for a date.

"Do you like it, Mom?"

"Well, of course, my son. It's wonderful," she said.

"Well, then…let's get it!" I said.

She protested, "It's too expensive, Dwayne." She was looking at the tags with the same sly look I remember from my boyhood.

I took her by the hands and said, "Mom, we can do this now. We can get anything you want."

My heart swelled with pride. I could finally say with conviction that she could have a shopping spree to end all shopping sprees. I sensed that while this was truly a "good day," not just in the context of her recent condition but of our entire life together. It wasn't "the two of us against the world" anymore. And it wasn't my mother against the world either. Her feistiness was fading. Just as I was finally entering a hard-earned era of success in my life and career, she was exiting the time in her life when she could have fully appreciated it, when it would have mattered most to her.

In the end, we bought something from nearly every single department: blouses, sweaters, shoes, coats, purses, jewelry. We had so many shopping bags that two employees had to help us carry them to the car. My mom was absolutely in her element. When we got home, she sat in the living room surrounded by her bags. She strategized about when and where she would wear each piece. "This will be perfect for brunch this weekend," she announced, pulling out a linen skirt and laying it across her lap. "Where is that pretty peach blouse? Oh, here it is. This will go with the flowered scarf."

That night, our second together, I replayed the day. It had been perfect. We were connected, laughing, and happy in each other's company. I was so grateful that I could spoil her. It's what I had been working towards for years. My mother had imagined it and now we were living it. And despite my earlier qualms, she seemed to be enjoying it completely. No drinking. No Jack. No drama. *This was all she needed,* I thought blissfully.

Still, I didn't sleep for most of the night. I would drift off only to startle awake. *What if Mom has fallen out of bed? Or down the stairs? Just because she hasn't woken up terrified doesn't mean it can't start anytime.* For the second night, I couldn't control my anxieties or stop myself from getting up, over and over, to check on her breathing, to make sure she was sleeping peacefully.

In the morning, I was so tired I could barely sort my thoughts well enough to get out of bed and get dressed. *How does Edweena do this? I'm a basket case after just a couple of days. How has she done this for months at a time?*

I started a mental list of things Mom and I could do today. *We could go to downtown Seattle and take a walk through the city's new art park. Mom will think some of the art is hilarious. This is just what she needs. Days filled with new experiences and moments of pure happiness.*

Terese was already up. I could smell coffee as I came down the stairs. She smiled when I came in, and we sat down together at the breakfast table, the morning paper spread out between us.

Mom walked down the stairs so quietly I didn't even hear her until she was in the kitchen.

"Morning, Mom. How'd you sleep?" I asked.

She didn't respond. She didn't even look at me. My mother seemed confused, pale, and distant.

"Would you like some coffee, Colleen?" Terese offered.

No answer, but she nodded, yes.

I stood up, took my mother's hand, and sat her down in a chair at the table.

"Are you okay, Mom?" I asked, still leaning close to her.

"Fine," she said quietly.

Her behavior reminded me of the way she would act when I was a little boy and had done something she didn't like. Mom's cold shoulder would humble all of us kids. But, now, she wasn't being deliberately aloof. She barely seemed aware of us. In a whisper I asked Terese to rely on her official nursing skills to evaluate my mother. I needed reassurance. Terese sat down and held my mother's hand gently.

"Are you hungry, Colleen?"

No answer.

"Would you like some breakfast?"

Still nothing.

Terese motioned for me to come with her to talk in the next room.

"I want to make sure she didn't have a TIA," she whispered. "I'll do a few strength tests and look at her pupils, but if it was a transitory stroke, we may not know."

"Okay," I said matter-of-factly, but I could feel my heart pounding. Mom had a history of mini-strokes and needed to be monitored carefully.

Terese returned to my mom's side and asked her to squeeze her hand. My mother did as she asked, while Terese looked at her pupils. "They seem fine," she said quietly to me.

"Do you know where you are, Colleen?"

"Of course. At my son's house," Mom replied, but still with little energy.

Terese stood up and moved next to me. "I think she's fine, just out of spirits," she said softly. "Maybe she's missing Edweena. If we put on some music we can see if that helps."

Terese is a big believer in the power of the senses to help us heal. She left the kitchen, and a few moments later the sound of Benny Goodman and his big band filled the room.

As I turned to ask Mom if she liked the music, she already seemed transformed. I could almost see her physically drawing in the sound. Her face loosened, color flowed to her cheeks, her posture straightened, her eyes sparkled and widened. She looked up at me and smiled. She seemed to come alive as she spoke up.

"I love this man!" she enthused. "Did I tell you I won a jitterbug contest to this song?"

"Well, let's see if you still have it in you, Mom."

I grinned, relieved and thankful, as I helped her stand up. She put her arms around me, arched her back a little, and wiggled her bottom, as though there were men lined up to take notice.

"Now son, I was also named best dressed at this dance, did I tell you that?" she asked, as I tried to keep up with her jitterbug. All of a sudden she could not stop talking, transformed into the chatterbox I knew and remembered. The medicine of music had put her in a better place and time.

I looked at Terese and saw tears rolling down her cheeks. I too started to cry, and I pulled my mother tight as we spun around the kitchen floor. I didn't want her to see my tears. This was our moment, and I would let nothing spoil it.

THE DIAGNOSIS

For two years after Mom's near-death experience at the diner, she continued to have plenty of good days, which only served to feed my denial about her condition.

As the CEO of a community of assisted living facilities, I had watched the scene play out dozens of times: Sons and daughters and loved ones locked in denial, refusing to believe that their mom or dad or spouse could possibly be suffering from Alzheimer's. They listen for any hint of reassurance from a trusted, long-time physician, who may not be apprised of all the symptoms by the patient or family members. They may not see their loved one regularly, or they may rationalize the behavior in the midst of their own very busy lives and worries.

Somewhere deep in my subconscious, I had to have known that this was coming, but like so many others I steadfastly held to my belief that Mom wasn't suffering from dementia. *Not MY mom*, I reasoned to myself. *She's just absent-minded, always has been. Perhaps her drinking is to blame, making her more confused and forgetful.* I created every possible excuse to postpone the inevitable, knowing that there was no definitive test, no pill, no cure, no way of diagnosing the disease until it progressed.

Still, Edweena and I searched out a geriatric specialist in Spokane. In my own mind, this would definitively answer the lingering questions, definitively rule out Alzheimer's as the cause of my mother's forgetfulness, her odd behavior. But when Edweena called with a report after Mom's evaluation, my rationalizations were immediately snuffed out and my worst fears confirmed.

I could tell from the tone of my sister's voice that it wasn't good news. As Edweena relayed the doctor's findings, I felt a rock in my gut. I had so hoped that I was wrong, but there could be no escaping this time: Mom had been "officially" diagnosed with Alzheimer's disease.

Looking back, I'm not sure why I felt shocked. I knew she was sick and, deep down, I knew what she was suffering from. Alzheimer's disease is the most common form of dementia. I knew it described her mental state and her prognosis. She was having difficulty processing information to a point that she was unable to function normally. Her behavior fit the signs of someone with a neurodegenerative condition.

But to actually have a doctor say it out loud, write it down, place it in a medical file—that made it profoundly real to me. I couldn't deceive myself any longer.

Edweena replayed the scene in the doctor's office: "The doctor says that Mom is in the early to middle stages of Alzheimer's disease. He said on the Reisberg scale of 1 to 7, Mom is a 3 to 4."

I said nothing in reply. Dr. Barry Reisberg developed his 7-point scale in 1980 as a tool to chart the impact of the disease. Stage 1 indicates a normal functioning adult, while Stage 7 is reserved for those who are unable to care for themselves at the most fundamental level. Mom's episodes definitively qualified her as Stage 3, with memory lapses that were noticeable and beginning to affect her ability to function independently at home.

As we talked over the details of the doctor's visit, we were both jolted into realizing how much Mom had changed in the six months since she had stayed with me while Linda and Edweena were on vacation. It was as if Mom had jumped off a cliff and was falling and failing at an accelerating rate. Sadly, Edweena and I had to agree that she was approaching Stage 4.

Edweena's voice cracked as she continued with the doctor's report. She concluded by stating the obvious: "The doctor also said—and made sure I understood—that Alzheimer's is a progressive disease. She'll only get worse."

Of course I knew that, but I still didn't want to accept it. It was too petrifying to even contemplate. I'd had a front row seat to the unrelenting chaos and pain that Alzheimer's can cause. Emotionally, spiritually, physically, the disease is ruinous, especially for the immediate family. In some ways, it is *most* difficult for the family because, at a certain point, the actual sufferer no longer cares about what is happening to them. The disease takes over and eventually leaves the person as a semi-permeable shell capable of recalling only dislodged, random fragments of memory. In the end, there are not even those memories to hold on to. For a spouse or son or daughter, there's just the flesh of the person you love, staring out into space, unblinking.

How many times had I seen family members visit their loved one, desperate to make a meaningful connection, only to be denied the smallest acknowledgement that they were actually in the room? How many times had I seen those family members leave in tears? Was it my turn to experience this torture?

I once heard a nurse describe Alzheimer's as "a force of nature." I suppose that's true, but when it's your own family member who gets the disease—when the person affected is the one who raised you, fed you, loved you, instilled you with the values and morals you apply to every life decision—it doesn't feel natural. It's as personal as it gets.

Mom's sick in a way she never would have wanted. Alzheimer's will crush her, will kill her spirit before it kills her body. It will crush all of us around her. And there's nothing we can do to stop it.

I still thought of my mom as I did when I was a boy, when she was the strongest person I knew, when I looked up to her for everything. She gave me the life I have. She made me the person I am. I owed her everything. When I imagined losing her, I reverted to a ten-year-old boy, when my sisters are leaving and my brother is leaving and she is all I have left. *What will I do without her? Who will I be?*

My only solace was my sense that this might be God's way of making her transition to the after-life easier. In my own spiritual way I had to speculate that the "Big Guy" had a plan, that he knew about Mom's fear of death and her abhorrence of the thought of ever being diagnosed with a terminal illness. It just wasn't something she could handle. Perhaps this way, her mind would slowly be sedated so she wouldn't have to contemplate the journey she was on. She wouldn't panic over what might happen and how and when it would manifest itself. She would just slowly and unconsciously move toward the fate that awaits us all.

If our memories are taken away, I wondered, *would our fears go as well?* As I faced the reality of my mother's future, I hoped and wished that were the case, though perhaps others might have seen it as an odd, almost childlike way to cope. Still, as we moved forward, it gave me some comfort knowing that Mom might be sheltered from her intense fear of death and the future ahead of her.

Idaho 1968
Granny and Me

There was a very important presence in our house when I was growing up: my grandmother, Agnes Gertrude Callahan. To me, Granny resembled the silhouettes that adorned so many Victorian-era brooches, with her long white hair pulled into a tight bun at the top of her head.

With Granny needing a place to make her home as a widow in the years after India's independence, she found her way to us. Perhaps my mom needed the most help and had the most open door. Granny came to live with us from the time I was small, and I look back on my time with her as a great gift.

She brought a calm constancy to our house, a commodity that my mother wasn't equipped to provide. Granny's routines and self-reliance, critical to survival in pre-war India, served us well as a struggling family in small-town Idaho.

Granny got up at 5:30 every morning and was back in bed by 8:30 each night. She drank a cup of tea at precisely 4:30 every afternoon, sitting always in the same chair in front of the living room window, Herman the dog at her side.

Granny offered me predictability. After my brother and sisters moved out, Granny became one of my closest friends. Nearly every day after school, she was there, at home, waiting for me with a Coke and a snack, usually a plate of cookies or brownies she'd baked, or on rare occasions a Twinkie or two. As she poured herself a cup of tea, she'd ask me about my day and always looked me in the eye as she waited for my answers. The genuine interest in what I had to say made me engage her in a different way than anyone else.

With Granny, I wanted to sound smart. I wanted to impress her. And because she had such a sharp wit, there was always an element of challenge in dealing with her. She asked me questions about my teachers and my friends and remembered the names of everyone from one story to the next. Interested in more than just the day-to-day happenings, she also asked me what I thought about the world. She wanted to know me. She made me feel older, more important that I would have otherwise.

She possessed that amazing gift of making me feel special. Before Christmas she'd ask me to "think about what you want on your next sweater."(She was a talented and quick knitter, a necessity in Depression-era India.) I'd say a cowboy or a car or a football, and there it soon would appear on a beautiful sweater hand-knit by Granny. I wish I still had one in a trunk somewhere.

I loved hearing her stories about life in India. It seemed like fantasy to a kid in Lewiston, Idaho, that someone in India might stumble upon a cobra coiled around the toilet. "What did you do, Granny?" I would ask breathlessly, pestering her for every detail. These exotic stories would impact me for the long-term, setting in motion an inner, almost insatiable desire to travel and see the world; so far, I've explored over eighty countries—and I've got more on my list.

Paradoxically, Granny had been a strict mother who had shown little emotion toward my mother and her other children, but the years had mellowed her by the time she was my daytime guardian and constant presence. Though she could still be a taskmaster, she was just as likely to laugh off a transgression that, once upon a time, would have warranted serious punishment.

Still, there were times when she was as strict with me as I imagine she was with my mom. Once, I told her to shut up when she teased me about having a girlfriend. I didn't mean it, but that didn't matter. There were just some things you didn't say to Granny. With a sudden strike reminiscent of those cobras she'd once known so well, she grabbed me by the earlobe—her patented move—and yanked me down to my knees.

"Don't you get cheeky with me!" Granny warned.

I howled. "Okay! Okay! I'm sorry!" Then I got the silent treatment until I apologized twice more.

Evenings would bring the three of us together—me, Mom, and Granny. Our bonding didn't take the romantic form of sitting on the porch, reading and sharing stories, as Mom's family did in India. Instead, we bridged our generation gap by watching television—the All-American pastime. We had a sixteen-inch, black-and-white Panasonic that tuned into the three networks plus a local cable station out of Lewiston. The picture was often filled with rolling static, and sometimes Mom would make me take the rabbit ears, extended with strands of tinfoil, and stand at odd angles so the image would focus. We all had our favorite shows: Granny loved panel shows like "To Tell the Truth" and "What's My Line?" I liked "Gilligan's Island" and "The Monkees," but really I'd watch almost anything. Mom was a huge fan of pro wrestling. Her favorite wrestler was a character named Dory Funk, Jr.

Every week, Mom sat between Granny and me as Dory Funk, Jr., successfully defended his National Wrestling Association World Heavyweight Title. "The cloverleaf! The cloverleaf!" Mom would scream, wanting to see Dory's trademark submission hold, the Texas cloverleaf, in which Dory would flip his opponent onto their belly, gather their legs, braid them together with his massive arms, and then lean slowly back, stretching the poor guy into a painful pretzel.

We went to see him live once in Lewiston. Mom got so excited when Dory made his way to the ring that she stood on her chair. "Dory, look over here!" she screamed, trying desperately to get his attention.

Dory was her perfect man: the man she could never have—famous, powerful, beautiful…unreal in every way.

To her, watching a wrestling match and connecting with its eccentricity was an escape from the monotony, the disappointments of daily life. She wanted to believe in crazy stuff. She'd pick up the *National Enquirer* and exclaim, "Look at this! JFK is alive and living in Peru!"

My mom certainly injected drama and fun into our home, but my grandmother contributed the simple joys that we all loved, too. Granny had lived her life with a steadfastness that carried her through many hard times with no parents, a large family, and the sudden loss of her husband. She had produced her opposite in my mother: a hellraiser throughout childhood and an unconventional adult and single mother whose unpredictability was both charming and maddening. I loved and depended on them both.

BREAKING POINT

Another call from Edweena. It had been a year and a half since we'd heard Mom's official diagnosis, and still my heart ached—for my sister, for Mom, for all of us.

Mom continued to live with Edweena, and my sister phoned me nearly every day, sometimes a couple times a day, just to vent. I didn't blame her. Maybe she was trying to say—to admit—it wasn't working to have her at home, but she didn't know how to. Or maybe none of her siblings were listening.

I had tried to help, but my efforts felt useless. Replacing Mom's caregivers didn't do any good. Mom would fire them or they'd quit out of frustration. The ones that did manage to tough it out didn't make much difference for Edweena. Mom's needs continued to overwhelm her. She was having a terrible time getting any sleep at night when she finally fell into bed or getting any work done when she got to her office. Nothing, it seemed, could relieve her exhaustion.

My worry about Edweena had started occupying as much of my thinking as my worry over Mom. I wondered what her breaking point was and I assumed she would reach it soon.

On this latest call, Edweena was telling me that Mom had crawled into bed with her and wouldn't stop talking. As a result, Edweena had only gotten two hours of sleep and had called in sick to work—again. Then she demanded Edweena get up and take her out for lunch.

Edweena told me that she had managed to nap for an hour that day, but when she woke up, she suspected that Mom had taken the opportunity to sneak some alcoholic drinks, undermining any rest she might have gotten.

In the past, Edweena had discovered bottles of vodka wedged in between the sofa cushions or tucked under Mom's bed, so I knew she wasn't imagining it. I talked to Mom for Edweena, a paternal role I'd fallen into, reminding my mother once again that she had promised to stop sneaking drinks. Mom sounded like a chastised little girl when she responded, "I'm sorry, my son. I know Edweena is upset. I don't know why she is so upset."

Just the week before, Edweena had to come home from work early because Mom wouldn't stop calling. She was yelling and cussing, telling her to "get your ass home right now!" But when I spoke with Mom later that day, she sounded fine. In fact, she was funny. Perfectly alert. She asked about the kids and seemed to be her old self. When Edweena got back on the phone, I realized I was reluctant to tell her, "Mom sounded pretty good," because somehow it might come across like an accusation.

The situation was unpredictable and erratic. Our dilemma was that Mom was still managing to have good days. She was still enjoying life, at least some of the time, though those times were becoming more rare. We were living the emotional roller coaster that is Alzheimer's.

Soon thereafter, Edweena and I got on yet another conference call with our sister, Linda, to try to figure out what to do. Mom's decline was real, and we could see it now. The bad days and neediness had become proportionally more than the "normal," okay days.

The option of institutionalized care was now on the table, and Edweena was the one who had finally put it there. She had dropped the idea on both Linda and myself several times, despite the fact that Mom had made it abundantly clear many times that she wanted to stay with Edweena. In fact, all our lives she had told us she would never tolerate going to "a home." At this point, we wouldn't think of openly discussing the option with her. She would go berserk.

Previously, Linda and I had suggested getting 24-hour in-home care for Mom, but it was hard to imagine how that would work. We doubted that Mom would let someone else care for her at night, when she was most frightened and confused.

We were going in circles, ending up nowhere. All we did was talk about Mom, but the talking wasn't making anything different or better. How could it? A person with Alzheimer's doesn't get better.

We had been avoiding the obvious, but now Edweena was worn out and worn down. It was clear we had no choice. In what would probably be the hardest decision we'd ever make, we decided to move Mom into a facility where she could receive around-the-clock care.

I knew for some time—before the official diagnosis, really—that there was the possibility we would end up at this point. I just never thought it would come so soon. But if we were to wait much longer, Edweena would be at real risk. She had lost so much already. For years, her world had revolved around our mother—to the point that she had abandoned her own needs, her sense of self. Now, everything she could call her own—her career, her health, her emotional well-being, her future—was in jeopardy. It was the domino effect of Alzheimer's, metaphorically knocking down everything and everyone in its path.

No matter how badly Edweena wanted to care for our mother, she simply couldn't. Mom needed to be monitored all the time. She needed expert care to make sure she got proper rest, medication, and nutrition. And there was no way Edweena could stop Mom's drinking (my mother routinely got her fix by calling a cab and sending the driver down to the liquor store to buy her vodka).

So with the facts clearly spelled out in our marathon phone call, we did what had to be done. There would be more phone calls, more research, and smaller decisions to wrangled over and made, but the waiting game was largely over. We would move my mom to an Aegis assisted living community.

We considered other facilities in Spokane so that she could be near Edweena, but we chose the Aegis property in Issaquah. It was a little farther away from my home than Aegis of Kirkland, but it was forty-five minutes closer for Edweena. As a bonus, Edweena's son, Derrick, oversaw the facility and Mom had always been very close to him. We knew it would be a comfort to her to have him near at hand.

Though we were fortunate that I was in the business of senior living, a fact that made it much less intimidating and easier financially than it would be for many other families, I soon discovered that nothing makes the finality of institutionalizing your sick parent any less gut-wrenching.

The room we chose looked out on a garden. Edweena started selecting the furniture: a firm bed topped with Mom's soft, old-fashioned quilt. We'd bring Mom's favorite table and lamp, her overstuffed rocking chair, and a couple of other comfortable loungers, as well as a television. Linda and Edweena found and framed old photos for her new room and they planned to hang the pastel floral prints from Mom's bedroom over her new bed. The idea was to make her new room feel like the home she'd lived in for years. Even though I knew all these steps well, I followed Edweena's lead. She seemed more at peace with the transition. More than any of us, she seemed to accept that the time has come for the move.

My sisters and I talked frequently during these few weeks of planning. We went over all the details, trying to imagine how we could make the move as peaceful as possible for our mother. But no matter how carefully we tried to anticipate her fears and confusion, I knew we couldn't avoid the trauma of the transition. I'd think about all I owed my mother and would wonder if there was any way she would understand why we had to do what we were doing.

We planned for Linda to come up from San Francisco for a week during the transition. We would each choose a few of Mom's belongings to keep as mementos. The only thing I cared for was a tall mirror with two little pictures showing some sort of Chinese ceremony inset at the top. It wasn't the material aspect of the mirror so much as the reflection of what it represented. It was a storybook of my youth.

I remember standing in front of that mirror as I marched off to fifth grade, taking a second and third glance, admiring my new terrycloth hoody. I remember putting on my football uniform and making mean faces in the mirror to practice my terror strategy. I remember standing in front of it as my mom snapped homecoming photos of my date and me in our splendid attire.

When I look at that mirror today I see what used to be. That mirror has so many different reflections. In it, I see the multiple facets of Collu, my mother. Our parents teach us to be the people we are. We pass their lessons onto our own kids. At the same time, we try to improve on what we've learned—the good, the bad, and the ugly—as we go along. I don't ever remember my father saying, "I love you, son." So I make a point of telling my children that I love them every chance I get. When I catch myself getting angry at daily trivia, I wonder if that's the way my dad was, if it's embedded in my genetic code to be like him. If I had known him better, I could say for sure.

But I know for sure what my mother taught me. She taught me to be proud and to dream big. She taught me to value each and every meal and to always look deeply into a person's eyes when I first meet them. She taught me the importance of leading by example and that education is a lifelong process. She taught me to be a vigilant, generous, grateful man and to laugh from the deepest part of my belly. She taught me how we should always stick together as a family and love each other no matter what.

And now I fear she'll never forgive me.

MR. GREENSHAW

When I was about eleven years old, I was called down to the principal's office at school. As I took the long walk down the empty school corridor, I wondered what I'd done to warrant being pulled from class. For the life of me, I couldn't remember violating any school rules and that made me nervous. When I got to the office, I was told that my mother was on her way to pick me up early. With no other details, I was forced to imagine what sin or crime I had committed. For Mom to actually leave work, I knew it had to be serious.

When she finally showed, she tried to stay calm, but I could see that she was stricken with worry and fear. She still wore her kitchen whites and her apron, lightly spattered with grease. She smelled of burgers and fries.

Apparently, Granny had tripped over Herman, our lazy, seven-year-old Pomeranian/Dachshund mix. Most days when I'd come home from school, I'd find the two of them on the couch watching "The Merv Griffin Show," Herman's head on Granny's lap and Granny scratching behind his ears. But on this day, Herman had been sprawled on the floor, in the wrong place at the wrong time.

We drove immediately to the hospital, where a doctor told us that the fall had broken Granny's hip. Due to her advanced age—she was eighty-one years old—my grandmother would be required to stay for several days before being transferred to a rehabilitation facility for at least two weeks. On hearing this grim news, Mom gripped my shoulder hard enough to make me wince.

When the doctor left, Mom turned away from me to look out a window. I stood there for a moment, before approaching her for a hug. That's when I realized that a tear was running down her cheek. She quickly wiped it away and put on a smile and told me not to worry. I nodded like I knew exactly what was going on, but silently I wondered why it was such a big deal. Granny broke her hip. She'd heal up and everything would go back to normal. But obviously, Mom knew different.

After her stint in rehab, Granny came home, but her needs were no match for our lifestyle. After only two days at home, it became clear that Granny required round-the-clock care, something we obviously couldn't provide, what with me in school and Mom working twelve-hour days.

So Mom had to send her mother to a nursing home. The facility was located in a nice neighborhood about fifteen minutes north of town, but the flat, gray building looked more like an industrial office park than a care facility. It was laid out in the shape of a cross, and the only nurses' station sat smack in the middle of the building, leaving the extreme ends isolated by corridors half-a-football-field long.

It wasn't a pretty place to visit but at least it was clean. Even so, the sharp smell of bleach constantly competed with the heavy odor of urine that wafted from the individual rooms into the halls. Typically, the doors to those rooms were left open, and as we walked the halls on our way to Granny's room, we couldn't help but peek into those private spaces. With some of them, it provided a nightmarish vision of what growing old could entail.

Many residents were physically bound to their beds. Some cried softly while others wailed at the top of their lungs, backs arching off their mattresses. Still others lay moaning, or humming softly, staring at the ceiling. The most horrific were those that lay silent, staring out the door. I'd catch their stares and see confusion or even panic in their eyes, and I'd quickly look away.

I remember wondering what these people had done to deserve their fate. The combination of the restraints and the screams and the smells gave the place a vibe that I identified with an insane asylum. It all seemed so cruel, barbaric, really, but I soon came to understand that the nurses had no choice. Without being physically bound to their beds, and without the better drug treatments and creative programs that are used in many facilities today, many of the residents who were still mobile but suffering from dementia would just get up and wander the halls. From there it was easy to see how they could make their way outside, down the street, and into traffic.

This was my first encounter with an elder care facility. At the time, I'm sure I would have thought it ludicrous if someone had told me that this would one day become my life's work, but today I have no doubts that my exposure to these residents had a profound effect on me. The whole place was like a way station for dying, abandoned, and lonely souls who had nowhere else to go and no one left in the world who cared. It was the only option for us, too—the only place close to home we could afford. I know it crushed Mom that we had no other alternative.

To her credit, Mom made the best of it. She visited Granny twice a day, every day, once before her shift in the morning and once after. Because she was there so often, she quickly made friends with everyone on the staff, from the head nurse to the janitor. Mom charmed them all, and within a week, Granny had been moved to a room next to the nurses' station, where she was constantly looked in on. Mom brought the nurses plates of cookies and slices of pie. She even introduced a couple of them to single men she knew.

Despite her heavy workload, my mother never missed a visit. Even on weekends, she spent two or three hours a day with Granny. As a result, I spent quite a bit of time there myself.

There wasn't much for me to do there. Of course, I spent time with Granny and told her about school and always gave her a report on what Herman was up to. We brought in a little black-and-white television so she could keep tabs on her game shows, and I would watch them with her. After an hour of sitting with her, though, I'd be itching to get out of my chair. Sometimes I went outside and played wall-ball, sometimes I'd even do my homework. But as I wandered the halls, I was always pulled toward one room at the far end of the hall.

A man lived in there, but every time I saw him, he was tied to his bed. He had long, wild hair, bone white and tangled, a stubbly beard and wide, round eyes. But they were kind eyes. I was drawn to him, I suppose, because he didn't scream or cry and it just didn't seem right that he should be tied down. Even if he was mentally impaired, I felt there should have been a better way for him to spend his time. He wasn't hurting anyone. He wasn't doing anything at all. He just lay there as if he were waiting for something, staring up at the ceiling or out his door. He caught my eyes more than once, and I got into the habit of checking in on him whenever we visited.

One day, after spending some time with Granny, I got restless and decided to make my rounds. Outside the white-haired man's room, I slowed for a look inside. He still lay on his back, his wrists bound by leather cuffs, yet he heard my steps and turned his head to catch my attention, smiling weakly. I smiled back and cautiously moved towards him, not quite crossing the threshold into his room. That's when the smell hit me; a dense putrid scent of urine and spoiled meat rolled out of his room and mixed with a sharp bleach smell that permeated everything. I was rethinking this idea of engaging him when his lips parted, showing his lack of teeth. He was barely audible when he mumbled, "Pillow."

Without entering his room, I made a visual search but didn't see any extra pillows. "Hang on," I said. "I'll get a nurse."

"No," he said. "Pillow."

I looked back down the long hallway, empty, and then again to the white-haired man who waited patiently.

"Please," he implored. "Help me."

"I don't see an extra pillow, sir," I explained.

He seemed to want to say something else, but he didn't. Instead, he shifted as much as his restraints would allow, leaning in my direction, and pleading with his watery, tired eyes. His look told me he wanted more than a pillow. He wanted out of his cuffs and out of that bed. He wanted to be treated like a man, with at least a shred of dignity. He wanted to live. Or maybe he just wanted to die.

"Pillow," he said, as he struggled weakly against his restraints.

I tried to step forward into his room, into that awful soup of sickness and age. But I couldn't. I was, suddenly, too scared.

I wish now that I could say that I helped him, that I marched into his room, found a spare pillow, and propped it under his head. I wish I could say we became friends and that he told me about his life. I wish I could say that I had the courage to go through that door and do the right thing.

Instead, I lowered my head and walked down that long hall to the nurses' station. The nurse on duty was working on a crossword puzzle and I told her that there was a white-haired man who needed another pillow. His room was all the way down on the right. She nodded at me but didn't move.

"He really needs a pillow," I said.

She looked up from her crossword and arched her eyebrows as if to say, "Excuse me?" Then she went back to her puzzle.

I shrugged my shoulders and started off towards Granny's room. Before I could get a few steps away, I once more felt the powerful tug to help but I rationalized that there was nothing I could do for him. I couldn't imagine facing that awful stench again. I returned to Granny's room and sat there brooding while Mom and Granny watched TV and ate Jell-O that had been molded into the shape of hearts.

It took me a few more visits with Granny before I finally summoned the nerve to visit the man's room again. I didn't want him to think I was a coward, so one day I mentally made preparations to march into his room, find him a pillow, and give it to him. When I finally made it down that long hallway, I peeked around his door only to find his room empty. Alarmed, I raced down to the nurses' station. "What happened to that man at the end of hall?" I asked.

"Oh, did you know Mr. Greenshaw?"

"Not really," I said. "But he asked me for help once."

"Mr. Greenshaw passed away two days ago. Very sad."

I couldn't believe it. I felt cheated and a deep sense of sorrow, and it must have shown on my face because the nurse gave me a sympathetic look and told me to stay put. She retreated into the shadows of the nurses' station and returned carrying a large cigar box.

"Look at this," she said, lifting the lid and pulling out a small stack of photographs. She placed them on the counter between us. I carefully picked up the top photo and saw a black-and-white image of a dashing dark-haired pilot in full flying leathers standing in front of a World War I bi-plane. He was looking off into the distance, holding his leather helmet in one hand and his pistol in the other.

"Wow," I said. "That's Mr. Greenshaw?"

"He flew for the British Royal Navy in World War I. He was an ace, which means he shot down a lot of enemy planes. Then he worked as a test pilot for the government and for Boeing, too. His wife died a few years ago. They never had kids so we're still waiting to see if there's someone to claim his effects. It's sad when there's no one left. It's the end of the family line."

"Yeah," I said, still looking at the image of Mr. Greenshaw. But it didn't make sense. How could this ace pilot and war hero end up tied down to a bed, alone, and begging for a pillow? More than anything, I wished I'd helped him. I felt guilty and ashamed.

"Thanks," I said to the nurse and handed the photo back to her.

After that, I wandered outside and waited for Mom to finish visiting with Granny. I just couldn't spend any more time in there. I had missed my opportunity to do the right thing for a poor, helpless old man. Now he was gone. I had chickened out and the guilt stayed with me for years. But a switch had been flipped. I no longer thought of him only as the withered and bedridden man I had avoided. To me, he was also a man who'd led a full, amazing life—a war hero no less. His life mattered—just like everyone's.

It took a long time to get his face out of my mind. But thankfully, mercifully, the image of the old man struggling against his restraints faded over time and I recalled the ace adventurer in the photograph. I don't know if anyone ever came for his things or if there's anyone else on this earth who remembers him now. But I do. And I still think of him from time to time.

That episode at the nursing home taught me another critical life lesson and proved a turning point in my life: Never again would I let myself shrink from fear. If my mind told me to do something, but fear threatened to hold me back, I would some-how find the strength and courage required to take action and do the right thing.

Part 3.

Sailing Away:
The Move

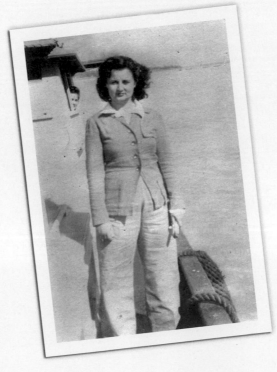

India, 1941: Colleen at age 18

Kennewick, Washington 1946: Newly married Colleen and Ed Clark

Kennewick, Washington 1956: Colleen, baby cousin, Edweena, Linda and Larry

MOVING DAY

Mom held onto Edweena's arm as they passed through the French doors and into a large foyer with high ceilings. Across the room, residents and family members chatted amiably in a parlor outfitted with elegant sofas and armchairs; others sat at the room's ornately carved walnut game table, playing bridge and enjoying a view that looked through large leaded windows and another set of French doors onto the sunny courtyard. The community was filled with warm inviting spaces, lovely gardens, and nature trails, all recalling a bygone era.

In the past, my mother enjoyed visiting Aegis communities with me, spending hours talking with guests, playing cards or Bingo. Not today.

She hadn't wanted to come with Edweena. She arrived confused and agitated, peering around suspiciously. Even though the sun was pouring through the windows and there were little kids happily running around outside, to her it might as well have been a haunted house on a dark and stormy night.

"I smell a rat," she said.

When I told her that this would be her new home, she cried and begged me to let Edweena take her home.

We had softened the news by telling Mom that this was a hotel that I had bought just for her, a luxury upgrade. I had to come up with some way to take the sting out of the fact that we were going against Mom's lifelong plea to never put her into a "home."

Telling her the "truth" wouldn't have served any greater purpose. If we'd been honest about the situation, it wouldn't have made sense to her and she would have made up information that did—however twisted. We had started doing the same thing.

"But I bought this hotel for you, Mom," I explained. "We've selected the finest suite for you and you'll have the entire staff available around the clock if there's anything you'd like."

She cast her gaze around again, looking up to the high ceiling and then through the front windows at the well-manicured lawn. I could see her eyes lighting up. Mom always loved to travel. She loved being pampered. The illusion that we had purchased her a special spa-hotel wasn't entirely untrue. I knew that she'd be well cared for by trained professionals: full-time nurses, talented chefs, a concierge, massage therapists, and a beautician. These were people who would see to Mom's every need. There would also be entertainment and companionship at the ready. Even though this wasn't an actual hotel, it might as well have been.

"And, for you, it's free," I said. "You don't have to pay a penny for it."

"Oh, my son, I am so proud of you. It really is a beautiful gesture. Thank you. Thank you. Where is your sister? Where is Edweena?"

"She'll come back soon," I said. Edweena and Linda had stepped out to get some last minute items for the room.

"Oh. And she'll take me home.... She'll take me home.... She'll take me home...."

Mom was mumbling now, repeating her greatest wish without realizing it. I started over, saying that I'd bought her a hotel and repeating the scenario, or a slight variation of it, several times over the next fifteen minutes. Each time she told me that she was going to haunt me until I got to the part about her own special VIP suite. Then her eyes would widen and she'd say how proud she was, only to slip back and ask yet again to be taken home. Each time she pleaded her case to go home, I felt a stab in my chest. It was torture. The little boy inside me was sobbing and begging for this moment to end. But on the outside I was smiling and nodding and smiling some more.

"But I bought this hotel for you, Mom," I pleaded again.

Guilt and anguish washed over me like a tidal wave. *This is what my mother has always dreaded, that her children would leave her.* The truth was: We weren't leaving her, she was leaving us.

My nephew, Derrick, the executive director of the community, showed up and soothed Mom by saying that he would be there with her every day. Derrick was like another son to her. Then my wife, Terese, my daughter, Ashley, my son, Adam, my niece, Alicia, and her boyfriend, John, and Linda and Edweena, all came to help ease the transition as well. Mom was surrounded by family.

Around seven that evening, after a full day of visiting with family and asking each of us if we could please take her home, Mom became tired and went silent. Edweena, who planned to stay at Aegis in case Mom needed her in the night, left to get a snack and make some calls. One by one, the others followed, until it was just Mom and me, sitting in silence in her room. A ray of golden-red sunlight peeked through and played on the opposite wall where I'd had an artist come and paint some giant butterflies. I thought for sure that Mom would like them since collecting them had been a favorite pastime of her childhood, but she hadn't noticed. The time passed slowly as the room got dark. I went to my mom and knelt beside her. The expression on her face remained blank, as it had been for nearly an hour. Her lips barely parted, forming a little O.

"Mom, I'm going to leave," I told her, "but Edweena will be back soon."

I took Mom's hand and squeezed it.

"I love you, Mom," I said, and kissed her on the cheek. I never imagined her this way, so fragile, so lost.

My mother didn't move. I let go of her hand and turned to leave.

"I'll never see you again," she said.

"Of course you will. I'll stop in tomorrow."

"No you won't," she said. She was getting agitated. "I want to go home NOW! Where's Edweena?"

"She's just making a phone call."

"Why are you doing this to me?"

"Because we love you," I said, my voice shaking. "Mom, we love you."

She bowed her head and looked at her hands, folded in her lap. I turned to go.

"Yeah, don't let the door smack you on the ass on your way out."

I should have taken offense, but instead a brief sense of joy came over me. Laughing to myself, I started to reply, but as I turned around I saw my mother's head still bowed, looking as sad and tired as ever. I slowly closed the door.

Edweena planned to stay for at least the first three days while Mom got settled. She also started to talk about moving and getting an apartment nearby. I tried to discourage her from making any snap decisions but I appreciated what this meant for her. She was clearly relieved to move Mom to Aegis, but it was still incredibly hard to give up caring for her. I remember thinking:

Today my mother and Edweena are saying goodbye to the life they've known together for so long.

Pride always ran strong within our family. Even though Edweena needed to reclaim her own life, the lingering guilt she felt for placing Mom at Aegis was crushing her. How many times had Mom sat one or another of us down and made us swear to her that we would never put her into a home? How many times had I heard this scenario over the course of my career in elder care? People simply run out of options. That point is different for everyone, but it almost always comes with guilt. This is never how anyone envisions the last years of a loved one's life. Edweena had reached her limit long ago, yet the pain of having done so was still acute. She was losing her companion in life—and her purpose.

Edweena only consented when she was on the brink of a collapse. At the time, simply saying "thank you" seemed so small a gesture for such an enormous sacrifice, and it still feels that way. But I know my sister and I know that she would have had it no other way.

Even so: Thank you, Edweena. You are an angel.

HALF A WORLD AWAY

After my mother graduated from St. Mary's, her time back in New Delhi was filled with friends, café life, and nanny jobs.

The Nazis, rattling for war with England, were half a world away in Germany, and my mother's family was certain that Gandhi and his Quit India Movement would never succeed. British rule would prevail. Nothing would change.

But, of course, the very next year, everything did change for the Callahans. My grandfather's sudden death required major adjustments. The estate was modest, by any measure, and there were no pensions nor life insurance to help pay the bills. Resourceful as ever, my grandmother wasted little time determining what she needed to do to support herself and the children who still relied on her. Within a year, she opened the Princess Marina, a seafood restaurant that catered to the British contingent.

My mother, Colleen, worked there, in any capacity she was needed. In the evenings, she sang for the dinner guests and, at age sixteen, had many admirers who came, hoping to catch a glimpse of the fit, dark-haired beauty, an Elizabeth Taylor lookalike who crooned the old standards with such verve. According to Aunt Joan, Colleen was fearless in front of a crowd, a natural performer. She'd get patrons going with "Roll Out the Barrel" and always finished the set with her favorite tune, a song that her father sang for her as a little girl, "Danny Boy."

Life would change for everyone on September 3, 1939, when England went to war with Germany. India's national and local governments, while supporting the allies and condemning Hitler, were not prepared to mobilize troops on the Allies' behalf. But as far as England was concerned, when England went to war, India went to war. The British Governor-General of India declared India's entry into the war without the approval of the Indian National Congress, and my mom was drafted into service with the Communications Corps of the Royal English Army.

Of course, everyone agreed that Hitler had to be stopped. It was a simple matter of right and wrong. And Mom was eager to do her part. Stationed in Calcutta, she learned Morse code and easily memorized all of the carrier signals for Allied and enemy aircraft. She once plucked out a stream of Japanese code from a seemingly meaningless transmission of static and isolated it. Apparently, within weeks of her training, she was tapping out encrypted messages twice as fast as anyone, man or woman, in the communications pool. She quickly rose through the ranks, eventually making sergeant.

Unfortunately, she still had problems with authority and was just as quickly stripped of her rank for insubordination. Still, thanks to her raw talent, the powers that be tolerated and even ignored her transgressions.

Once, she ignored the curfew and subsequent lockdown so that she could attend a local dance. She was reprimanded and confined to her barracks, but a week later, when she heard that there was another dance with contests scheduled, she violated her probation and climbed over the wall, her ball gown tied around her waist. She lost the jitterbug contest but was crowned "best dressed."

It was at one of these dances that she met Ed Clark, an American G.I. who worked as a supply sergeant. Thanks to his position and rank, Ed was a very popular man. Get on his good side and a world of rationed supplies opened up to you. Colleen and her best friend set out to befriend Ed with the specific purpose of securing essential goods: nylon stockings, cigarettes, chocolate, and American chewing gum—a real treat for the girls, who had never chewed gum in their lives. Ed was taken with Colleen from the start. But despite the fact that he was rugged, handsome, and well dressed, Colleen was initially repelled by Ed's brusque cowboy manner. She maneuvered her friend Dolly into dating Ed to keep their supply lines open, but Ed never let Colleen forget that he was interested.

By contrast, Colleen's attention focused on the love of her life, Lucas Carter, a medic who had recently returned home to New York. Their short romance had lasted for only a handful of dates before Lucas was reassigned back to the States. But before he left India, Lucas professed his love and promised Colleen that, when the time was right, he'd send for her. According to Mom, he was a tall blond, with dark blue eyes and a swimmer's lean, graceful physique. He was a wonderful dancer and a true gentleman. Better yet, he was a college graduate who had planned to complete medical school. And he was ready to get married and start a family as soon as possible. In short, he was perfect.

They corresponded for nearly six months and Lucas sent hundreds of dollars in cash. Dutifully, my mother tucked it all away in a cigar box for her future trip to America. But then the letters stopped coming, just like that, the poems and the promises gone. She sent letter after letter to no effect. Finally, broken-hearted, she gave up.

A few months later, Ed got down on one knee and begged Colleen to go out with him. "You're the prettiest thing I've ever seen," he told her. "I'm going to die right here on this spot if you don't go to dinner with me."

How could she say no? She was still suffering from her loss of Lucas Carter, but she wasn't about to let a little thing like a failed romance spoil a potentially good time with another good-looking, well-dressed American G.I., especially if there were desirable gifts thrown into the bargain.

It turned out that they were well matched in temper, humor, and energy. In the long run, though, they were probably too much alike to last.

I don't think my mother ever fell completely in love with Ed Clark, at least not in way that she had with Lucas and, later, Art, the traveling salesman. But the war was winding down, as was British rule, and the country was going to be turned upside down.

On my mother's twenty-first birthday, my grandmother took her aside for a heart-to-heart. "You must find a way to get out of this country and go to America," she told her daughter. "Get married. Start your life in a new world."

"But this is where you are, my family, my friends, everyone," Colleen protested. "I can't leave you. What would happen to you? What would I do there in America?"

"I don't know," Agnes said. "But you must think of your future. There's no future for you here."

Colleen reluctantly agreed. The atmosphere was becoming downright hostile towards British nationals. So when Ed finally proposed, Colleen didn't hesitate. They married in a military ceremony at the base chapel in Calcutta on April 7, 1946. As their ceremony concluded, a full Honor Guard formed an arch of sabers under which they proudly strode arm in arm. And as they passed the final soldier, he brought the flat of the sword down and swatted her on the bottom.

Ed planned to re-enlist, but he came down with a strain of tropical malaria that left him bedridden and unable to continue his military service. It was decided that the newlyweds would return to Ed's home in Washington State so that he could recover at home with his family and friends. Colleen wanted to travel by plane—it excited her—but she learned that the military would pay for the trip only if they traveled by sea. She was petrified of the open water, but there was no other way. She resigned herself to a long sea voyage.

They boarded *The Marine Panther,* a medical corps vessel out of Calcutta and bound for San Francisco, and settled in for what would be a twenty-eight-day passage. My mother referred to it for the rest of her life as "that awful trip."

Before leaving, she requested that her family not see her off at the dock. She didn't want an overtly emotional goodbye. Instead, she chose to see each of her brothers and sisters individually in the days leading up to the departure. Only Granny actually saw her off at the docks, so distraught over her leaving that she could barely manage to speak.

"We'll see each other again," my mother promised.

"You were your father's little girl," her mother said. "But you were mine too. Never forget where you came from and who you are. Your family loves you forever. You are an exceptional young woman and you will always be in our thoughts."

And so, with a mix of sadness and excitement, Colleen boarded the ship, went to the rail, and waved a final farewell to her mother, to India, and to the only life she'd ever known.

WHERE'S HOME?

Today was one of those "people" days at the office. Of course all of our work is about people—those we serve, those we encounter, those we work with every day. But sometimes we have a day that is all about human beings and their growth. On this day, my tasks ranged from considering a creative request for a raise and new responsibilities to having a conversation with a key staff person who needed to be let go in spite of efforts on both sides to make it work. The highlight of the day, though, was a formal meeting with Ashley—as formal as it can get with your daughter—to talk about her career possibilities.

At the time, Ashley was twenty-two years old and absolutely glowing with youthful energy. She would always look me in the eye and smile and it gave me goose bumps. She was—and still is—beautiful, funny, and razor sharp.

I got home feeling tired but full from the many meaningful conversations of the day and looking forward to sitting down to a home-cooked meal. That's when the phone rang.

"Hello?"

"Hi, Dwayne, it's Derrick. I'm with Gram."

My heart was suddenly in my throat. "What is it? Is she okay?"

"She is, but she's really upset. I came in to try to calm her down, but I wasn't able to help. I'm sorry. I tried."

"What's the matter with her?"

"She's screaming. She's scared. She wants to go home. She wants to see my mom. She thinks we've kidnapped her. She keeps repeating the phone number. That's what she's doing right now, just repeating the number over and over again. And she's crying."

"Okay," I said. "I get it. I'm on my way."

I hung up the phone and looked at Terese, and we both sighed.

"Can I go with you?" she asked, putting her hand on top of mine.

"No," I said. "I won't be long."

"You don't have to do this alone. I'm ready to go with you," she said as she handed me a chicken leg to tide me over until I got back home.

"Thanks," I said. "But it's okay. I'll call."

I spent the next fifty minutes navigating the remains of Seattle rush-hour traffic. The good feelings of the day drained away. I felt trapped, trapped in my car, trapped in traffic, trapped in a reality I couldn't face. I wanted to be there for Mom. This was my chance to do what was right and what she needed. It was my chance to give her what so many older people don't have—someone who cares. That haunting image of the ace pilot Mr. Greenshaw asking for a pillow floated into my consciousness. I wanted to help, but I also wanted to avoid the pain.

Then my mind floated to another image—the cozy house where my mother had lived with Edweena, where the two of them had made so many memories. When Mom got really worked up, she'd just repeat their phone number over and over. How does this disease pick and choose the things it takes and the things it leaves behind? For Mom, it always led back to Edweena.

No matter how frequently Edweena visited, when she left, Mom invariably would realize that she wasn't going "home" and would throw a fit. She'd scream for Edweena and threaten to leave. She'd accuse the nurses of holding her hostage. My sister could barely handle this emotional onslaught. When my mom cried inconsolably, begging Edweena to take her home, I watched my sister crumble. A few times, she even seemed ready to relent.

This past weekend when Edweena had visited, Mom acted great, the best she'd ever been. She commented on how clean the building was and even said that she liked the staff. But once Edweena left, everything went back to the way it had been, maybe even worse. As a way of soothing her and keeping her occupied, we had allowed Mom to sit in Derrick's office while he made phone calls, but when he needed to do other things, Mom would get possessive and needy.

When I finally arrived, Derrick and the head nurse greeted me at the door. They were both smiling as I approached. Derrick took a step forward.

"She's fine now," he said. "She's totally calmed down and she's making jokes with anyone who walks into her room. We told her you were on the way and she mellowed right out."

"Go on home," I said to Derrick. "And thanks for coming all the way out here after hours."

"No problem," he said.

With that, I walked to Mom's room. At the door, I took a deep breath and knocked.

"Mom, it's Dwayne."

"Come in, my son," she said.

She was sitting in her recliner, watching "Wheel of Fortune" on her little color television and snacking from a small bowl of popcorn.

"Oh, I wasn't expecting you," she said. "Pull up a chair. How are you?"

"Good," I said. I pulled the desk chair over so I could sit right next to her. "How are *you*?"

"Me? Oh, I'm fine. Just watching the show. They were making a fuss before, but everything is just fine now."

She looked at me, tousled my hair, and added, "Now that you're here."

My sense of relief faded when I heard the line, "I'm just happy to see you, my son. I've been meaning to talk to you about something."

"Sure, Mom," I said.

Mom turned and looked directly at me. Her eyes were set and remarkably clear as she spoke.

"My son," she said, almost apologetically, "I spoke with your sister and we both agree that it's time for me to go back home."

"Oh. You spoke with Edweena?"

"That's right. Another thing, my son. I know this isn't a hotel."

I sighed. "Yeah, Mom, you're right. It's not."

Since we'd moved her into Aegis I'd never seen her this focused and clear-headed. I was sure she hadn't spoken with Edweena, so I knew that element of her statement was a fantasy. Still, I wanted to take advantage of her being so present and sharp. My first thought, as ridiculous as it seemed, was to take her to dinner so that we could have some time together like we used to.

"Derrick told me that you had a good breakfast the other day," I said, changing the subject. "He said that you finished a big plate of eggs and bacon."

"Oh, and when did he tell you that?"

"Yesterday."

"I didn't eat breakfast here yesterday. I wouldn't eat the food that comes out of that kitchen." Mom had a life-long inclination to never compliment someone else's food, so it didn't surprise me that she'd make a crack about the food here.

She was about to say something else when she stopped suddenly and looked around the room. She seemed surprised, as if she'd just forgotten something important. An expression of utter confusion washed over her face. She put her head in her hands and started to cry. I reached out to give her a gentle embrace, but before I could, she pushed me away.

"Why won't you let me go home? Why are you doing this to me? You are my son. MY SON! You are supposed to do what I say! You're supposed to honor me and love me! I'm your mother! YOUR MOTHER!"

"I do love you, Mom. That's why I'm here. Please," I pleaded. "Everything will be fine."

But she wouldn't stop sobbing. "Why is this happening to me? You're supposed to love me . . . Where's Edweena? I must go home now!"

"I know," I said. "I know."

I turned on the TV and slowly she stopped crying and nodded off to sleep. I sighed in relief and rose to leave. But as I tiptoed out of her room, she stirred.

"This isn't a hotel, my son," she said, without opening her eyes, and then she went back to sleep.

Outside, the night air was cold and cut through my nylon windbreaker. There weren't any stars in the sky, just an inky blackness.

Once in the car, I rolled the windows down to pull in the chilly blast of nighttime air. The air mixed with the music from the car radio and I began to feel something like relief. Even though Mom was having her troubles, I felt fulfilled from doing my part—the human part, not just the financial part that had been so much of my role up until now. As hard as this was, it was also profoundly rewarding.

I was in the trenches now, where I belonged. I remembered how diligent Mom had been in her visits to Granny. Twice a day, every day, she made time for her mother. It seemed impossible to live up to that. I rationalized that Mom's and Granny's circumstances were different, but it didn't take the guilty sting away completely. I understood that visiting Mom was something I needed to do while I still had the chance. This was my duty as her son, my honor.

This was the time to do whatever I could for her.

That Awful Trip

Moving my mother to Aegis was wrenching and full of the same high-level drama that had marked other turning points in her life. But this would be her last move and it held no sense of the promise that others had.

Her most momentous journey had been the one that had taken her to America. I've always loved that image of her on the open sea, bound for America with little more than a few suitcases packed with all her worldly possessions and a heart full of hopes and dreams.

She was seasick virtually every day, so much so that she lost fifteen pounds. Her new husband, Ed, was stowed away in a medical cabin, where he was treated for the malaria that had set in. The doctors were very strict about visiting times, so Colleen had almost no contact with her new husband during that dreadful month at sea.

Upon docking in San Francisco, Ed was transported directly to the hospital and admitted to a critical-care ward where he was heavily sedated to deaden the pain and given intravenous medications to treat his fever and combat the illness. Colleen wasn't even allowed to see him. At one point, they couldn't even tell her which wing of the hospital he'd been taken to. She was suddenly, utterly alone, a feeling she had known at St. Mary's, but here it was much worse. The government provided a dingy hotel room for her in a downtown district not far from the seedy waterfront. At night, the blast from the foghorn woke her up once every hour.

My mother's first days in America must have been the loneliest of her life. She was cut off from everything she knew, most significantly the circle of friends and family that had always surrounded and buoyed her. From one minute to the next, she didn't know whether her husband was dead or alive and if she'd find herself abandoned in a strange country, fueling her lifelong fear of being alone.

Everything about San Francisco seemed to overwhelm her. Despite being strong-willed and adventurous, my mother was stranded in a foreign land, with no sense of the local culture and with no one to turn to for help or friendship. It was cold and rainy, and a dense fog swallowed the city. She spent two full days locked in her room, questioning her choice to come to this God-forsaken place. Hunger finally forced her onto the street, where some helpful strangers took pity on her and helped her to a diner. After a few more days, Ed finally regained consciousness.

Colleen went to his bedside and begged him to help her get out of the city. Fortunately, Ed was bound for the Fort Lewis Army Hospital in Tacoma, Washington, where they'd keep him under observation for six to eight weeks to make sure the infection was contained. Ed called home and arranged to send his new bride to stay with his parents in Kennewick, Washington, a tiny town in the southeastern part of the state. Based on the one-half of the conversations she'd heard, Colleen believed the reception might be a chilly one, but she didn't care. She just wanted to get the hell out of San Francisco.

The train ride north was magical. Compared to India's ancient unknowableness, the America rushing past her window was exactly what my mother had hoped for. This was the fresh, wide-open frontier of the New World. She spent much of the trip glued to her window, watching it all go by. She also met a number of friendly people along the way and noticed that her accent drew the attention of almost anyone within earshot.

One man in particular, a train porter, stuck in her memory as being helpful and friendly. He was a short, elderly African American with a genuine smile, bright eyes, and beautiful hands with long, elegant fingers. He wore a spotless uniform, perfectly fitted and creased, and he removed his cap and bowed when he first met Colleen. "My name is Washington, but I'd be pleased if you called me Wash. Everyone does."

Where most people barely regarded him, Colleen looked Wash in the eye, thanked him warmly, and confided to him that she was new to the country.

"Well, we'll have to make sure you're treated right, then. We wouldn't want you to come away with a bad impression of us," Wash said with a wink.

Wash impressed her tremendously, and they instantly struck up a friendship. He reminded her of the servants back at home in India, always genuine, friendly, and helpful, not because they were being paid but out of warmth and kindness. For the duration of the trip, Wash made sure that Colleen was comfortable.

My mother considered Wash to be the first true gentleman she'd met in America. "He treated me with dignity," she recalled. So many of the stories she told me as a child concluded with the same moral lesson: Treat people right and they'll treat you right.

When the train finally arrived, Wash insisted that Colleen allow him to carry her bags from the platform into the station proper. As she said goodbye to him, Colleen emptied her purse of all the change she'd accumulated since her arrival, and deposited it in Wash's cap. He bowed to her and thanked her profusely.

"It was an honor to make your acquaintance," Colleen said.

"The honor was entirely mine, ma'am," Wash replied, before bowing a final time and turning on his heel.

At the station, Colleen, excited and nervous, waited for her new in-laws. She waited and watched and wondered if Ed's parents had been given the proper information. Maybe they were expecting her to come in on a different train? What other reason could there possibly be for them not being on time to meet her? Colleen settled in to wait.

An hour later, another train unloaded, and her hopes rose again. Again, passengers filled the station and the echoes of joyous reunions rang through the building. For a second time, Colleen watched as travelers were welcomed with hugs and tears. There were soldiers home from the war, students home from school, and tramps who had no home, skulking silently away. But again, there was no sign of the Clarks. When she found herself sitting in the empty station for a second time, she began to worry.

She checked with the ticket taker to see if there were any other trains arriving from San Francisco on that day, and when she learned that hers was the only one, she decided to call them.

No answer.

She sat back down and continued her vigil. Another train unloaded and then another. She called after each train pulled into the station, but no one came to pick her up. The afternoon faded to dusk. Was she once again all alone in America?

The Clarks finally walked into the station lobby, three hours after Colleen had arrived, but she didn't see them. Due to the lateness of the day, she was sitting all alone in the station, so they were easily able to spot her. My mother looked up to see a neatly dressed couple looking down at her—but with no smiles on their faces.

After curt hellos and no apologies or explanations for leaving their new daughter-in-law waiting half the day, my paternal grandmother apparently announced with disappointment, or possibly suspicion, "I thought you'd be wearing a sari," a flowing Indian robe.

"Why would I do that? I am a British subject, Mrs. Clark," my mother remembered replying, without any meekness or deference.

That first meeting was a miserable moment for my mother, an indicator of the long months that lay ahead for her.

Wordlessly, the Clarks gathered Colleen's few belongings, packed her into their car, and took her to their home in Kennewick, Washington, which, along with Richland and Pasco, made up the Tri-Cities of southeastern Washington.

This was her new family. Big Ed Clark was a successful rancher and real estate owner, while Laura taught the fourth grade. They were stern frontier people who'd lived through the worst of the Great Depression. They spoke only when something needed to be said and didn't smile or laugh easily. In my mother's eyes, Ed and Laura Clark were hillbillies. She was a spoiled princess in theirs. Their opinions of each other wouldn't change much over the years to come.

The Clarks lived in a relatively nice home, but the arid, plains climate was a dramatic difference from what Colleen had known in India. She was given a guest room of her own and tried to acclimate herself to this new world. But it was a challenge from the start. Everything was different for her now.

The Clarks barely spoke to Colleen, and when they did the topic rarely strayed from Ed's condition. He was still in the hospital at Fort Lewis, a four-hour drive from Kennewick. When the Clarks announced plans to visit him at the end of the first week, Colleen was over the moon. Yet her excitement was met with stony silence, something she didn't understand. She'd done nothing but be polite and quiet. She wanted to scream at them for being so rude. But she held her tongue and sat straight in her chair at every meal.

What Colleen didn't know and only learned years later is that the Clarks had planned for their son to marry another woman, his high school sweetheart, a blonde and blue-eyed beauty named Sabrina Logan. Sabrina's parents were great friends of the Clarks, and they'd spent many nights playing bridge and talking about their children. Together, they dreamed of how wonderful a couple Ed and Sabrina would make. Colleen had unwittingly played the part of the spoiler. She never had a chance with the Clarks.

On the first trip to Tacoma, Colleen and the Clarks learned that Ed was finally getting better after nearly two months of being deathly ill. The doctor was convinced that Ed could return home within two weeks, though it actually took another month.

Colleen passed the time reading whatever books she found in the house or small store in town and wandering the streets and vast grassy fields.

When Ed finally returned, his presence lightened the mood to the point that his parents actually seemed to enjoy Colleen. They visited neighbors, went shopping together, and ate out often. Everywhere they went, there was someone who wanted to shake Ed's hand and thank him for his service. But even as she was finally able to enjoy life as a new bride, Colleen knew their honeymoon period would be over very soon. Her morning nausea and sudden need to take afternoon naps forced her to confront the fact that she was pregnant.

Colleen was finally being viewed as a member of the family and Laura attended her with genuine care. But the cramped surroundings and the utter lack of privacy in the Clarks' home took their toll.

My strong-willed mother sat Ed down and told him that it was time to move out of the family home. Ed didn't understand. He explained that they couldn't afford a house while he was still looking for work. But Colleen knew that the Clarks owned several houses in the area. They could ask his parents for one of those homes. It would be temporary and they'd pay rent, but at least it would be theirs, she argued.

After more discussion with Ed and displeasure from his parents, the couple finally got their first place, a home of their own. My older brother, Larry Ray Clark, was born on November 22, 1946. November 22 was also the birthday of my maternal grandmother, Agnes, and, later, mine.

Four years later, Colleen went into labor with Edweena. Laura came over to watch three- and four-year-old Linda and Larry, and Ed piled Colleen into the car and rushed to the hospital. As they got close, Ed noticed that it was 11:45 p.m. Instead of continuing into the parking lot, he unexpectedly pulled the car over, turned the ignition off, and calmly folded his arms.

"What the hell are you doing?" Colleen demanded. "We're still ten blocks from the hospital, for Christ's sake!"

"Let's just sit tight here until midnight. It's only another few minutes."

"Are you out of your mind?" Colleen screamed as she felt the pinch of another contraction.

"They'll charge us for a full day if we go in there right now. We don't have health insurance. Just sit tight and we'll go in at midnight. It's not like you're going to pop right here and now."

My mom went berserk at Ed's spendthrift plan. She scratched at his face, got a good grip on his shirt instead, and ripped part of it right off of him, shredding it into strips. But still, they waited until midnight before Ed restarted the car and drove the rest of the way to the hospital.

My father was a good-looking hometown war veteran, with his genius IQ. He should have had an easy time of it. But he didn't.

He was restless and a wanderer. The yoke of his growing family didn't help.

Later in life, when my mother would retell the story of Edweena's delayed entry into the world, it would typically be as a humorous anecdote. As we soon discovered, though, it was a harbinger of things to come.

"I THINK I'M LOSING MY MIND"

A year after Mom's move, Aegis of Issaquah held its annual community bash, the biggest event of the summer. This year we planned a luau, complete with a Hawaiian barbecue, a ukulele player, and a trio of young hula dancers in grass skirts. We burned Tiki torches and wore leis over flower-printed shirts. All of the residents and their families were encouraged to attend. Kids played and danced and ran around, with around 150 people crowded onto the lawn. It also marked the biggest gathering of our family since Mom had come to live here.

I prayed that this would be a good day for my mother and that she would enjoy all the attention—as she still did on occasion. She was living in the general assisted living wing, not the other side reserved for people with full-blown Alzheimer's disease. Was that for her benefit, or for ours?

She had been dealing with some depression, a common occurrence with Alzheimer's patients. I think, on some level, she had finally realized that this was her new residence, though she continued to ask for Edweena and repeated her wish to return home on a daily basis. We all hoped that the impromptu family reunion would spark her love of parties and buoy her spirits.

Unfortunately, as is the case with many Alzheimer's patients, she didn't respond well to all the stimuli. The music, the people, the family, the smells, the movement—it was all too much for her. She started out strong, but quickly became overwhelmed.

So instead of a happy occasion, the bash quickly turned into something grim, almost like a wake. Mom was alternately confused, unhappy, and forgetful. Everyone who tried to interact with her noticed it.

Despite the distraction of the day's happy festivities, Mom's worsening condition was the main topic of conversation for all of us. The year before, we'd seen her go from a confused older person dealing with gradual memory loss to mounting changes and limitations that made daily living more of a struggle. Now it was clear that she had entered a whole new stage of Alzheimer's, and yet again we weren't prepared to accept her rapid decline—the emotional swings, the delusions, the repetitive statements, and other distressing symptoms that marked the advancement of Alzheimer's.

Being there together, collective witnesses to this decline, forced us to hold each other accountable to the fact that it was time to live according to her true reality, not our wishful thinking.

Late in the afternoon, she seemed to perk up a little so I went over to her. Edweena was sitting with her as well.

"Hey Mom," I said.

She looked at me, searching my eyes for a second. I wasn't sure if she recognized me.

"Are you okay, Mom?" I asked. "What is it?"

She huffed, clearly frustrated.

"What is it, Mom?" I asked again.

"I think I'm losing my mind," she said.

Such a simple statement, but it hit my heart with the power of a gunshot. This was not the throwaway line people say when they're angry or feeling overwhelmed or attempting to explain away memory lapses. This was my mother admitting, saying out loud though in a near-whisper, what had been going on inside of her for so long now.

Six little words, so deep and powerful, coy and soft: "I think I'm losing my mind."

She was alert and awake, telling us that she knew she was going crazy. She was sailing into a fog, leaving us behind on a one-way journey, and it felt like we were saying goodbye. There was only one destination possible.

I could feel it. *My mother is entering a new chapter where she will completely lose her sense of herself, and we'll lose her—the person we've known. Her hand is slowly being pulled out of ours.*

Edweena and I glanced at each other, then back at Mom. We both put our hands on hers.

"No, you're just fine," Edweena reassured her. "You just relax and have some fun."

I put my hand on Mom's shoulder, rose from my seat, and wandered over to the buffet. I couldn't let go: *She's losing her mind and she knows it.* I put a few things on a plate and sat down at a lone picnic table. A few minutes went by before a pair of couples approached my table and sat without introducing themselves or even acknowledging me. Fine, I thought. The table was very long and they had their end and I had mine. I didn't feel like small talk.

I couldn't help but overhear their conversation: They were family members of a current resident and they were talking about Aegis, about the care their loved one had received. Mostly, it was positive, but then, one of them made a remark regarding the unfairness of a recent rent increase. Another commented on an employee who had been short with her on the phone. I kept my head down and felt, suddenly, like a spy.

Of course, if they had known I was the head of the company, they would never have said these things. I wasn't sure if I should simply leave or just stay there and listen. I wanted to hear the unfiltered feedback, but I didn't want to eavesdrop either. It made me angry to be pulled in two different directions. I just wanted to be Mom's son that day, not the person in charge. I started to get up from my seat when, as if on cue, Derrick approached and introduced me to everyone at the table.

"This is Dwayne Clark. He's the CEO of the company," Derrick said.

I looked up and tried to smile. I felt like an ass, and I'm sure it showed. Surveying the expressions around the table, I saw that everyone was working on a reply or was too mortified to move. Then the image of my mom, the idea that she was so very sick, hit me like a boomerang in the back of the head.

"Excuse me," I said.

I went to the bathroom to wash and clear my head. I looked into the mirror, looked deeply into my own eyes, seeking out some inner wisdom, anything that might give me strength. I felt lost and tired and I just wanted to be home, under the covers, with the phone unplugged. I wanted to be unconscious, removed from everything. I couldn't take it anymore. Mom was losing her mind.

Then I thought of my son, Adam, and my daughter, Ashley, who were both at the party. It came to me that just seeing either one of them smile or laugh would help. I left the bathroom with a new purpose and, sure enough, they were both there, leaning over Mom, their grandmother. All three were engaged and, despite Mom's general bad mood, in that moment they'd made her smile. It was such a beautiful sight to me that I felt a warm rush of good feelings. Ashley looked up and smiled in my direction.

I smiled back but stood my ground. I didn't want to ruin this picture: my children and my mother.

As the day progressed, Mom became agitated and angry and finally wanted to go back to her room. She was fed up with everyone. "All fakers," she snarled. Edweena wheeled her away and everyone suddenly felt the absence. There was little more to say after that, and in a short while everyone was getting ready to leave. Adam came to me to say goodbye.

"I feel so bad about Gram," he lamented.

"I know, it's really sad," I agreed. "I'm glad that you were here, though. It's all about the moment for her," I reminded him.

Later, after everyone had gone, I went to Mom's room. Edweena was there, sitting on the edge of her bed, stroking Mom's hand and talking about old times. Her eyes were bright, and she smiled as I approached.

"Hello, my son," she said.

"Hello, my mother," I offered back.

"I really liked those hula dancers," she remarked.

I sat across from Edweena and joined in the reminiscing. But my thoughts wandered between our long pauses in conversation. I thought about this disease and how insidious it is, how after all that had happened earlier, here she was, totally normal, relaxed, her old self. Part of me knew that I should cherish this moment. But I couldn't. I felt such rage.

This disease couldn't be nastier, yet I knew it wasn't actually evil. It doesn't care one way or another, just as a tornado doesn't care which house it destroys, just as a butterfly doesn't care which flower it lands on, just as an ocean current doesn't care where it takes the lone survivor's raft. This disease is simply a force of nature. An unpredictable, unfair, and unrelenting force of nature. My mother was sailing away.

I stayed there with my sister until Mom fell asleep. After that, Edweena and I sat on the edge of the bed for a long time, just watching Mom, not saying anything. Finally, she seemed at peace.

"We can leave now," Edweena said.

I couldn't move. I was still fixated on Mom's sleeping face. Finally, my sister came over to me and grabbed me by the arm.

"Let's go now," she said.

I stood up but didn't move. I wasn't feeling sad or guilty or remorseful. I was just very, very tired. It felt like mourning, because even though Mom was lying there in front of me, alive and breathing, there was a part of her that was gone. And such a fantastic part of her—her humor, her wisdom, her larger-than-life, over-the-top personality.

"It's okay, Dwayne," Edweena whispered. "We can go now."

MAN OF THE HOUSE

I was a preteen when I discovered how the other half lived.
Gale Wilson, one of our school's popular kids, invited me to
his house to hang out. He lived on Sunset Drive, up on the hill
in the newer part of town where the mill executives of Potlatch
Forest Incorporated and other important personages of Lewiston lived; I thought of them as the country club set.

I had never been up on the hill. It took only a few minutes riding my bike to reach his house, and when his mother opened the
door, she was wearing an apron. The house smelled of cookies.
"Gale's downstairs with his dad," she said. I walked past the
perfectly dusted furniture and thought: *Wow, they have
a downstairs!*

I descended the steps and found Gale and his father in the well-furnished family room sitting in two comfy chairs, near a fire
blazing in the fireplace and on either side of a big barrel of walnuts. They were cracking the nuts together. His dad was smoking a pipe and wearing a sweatshirt emblazoned with a college
logo—both signs to me that this was indeed the All-American
family. I looked around the room, which was filled with pictures
of the family's ski vacations and annual trips. I was speechless.
I felt as if I'd just walked into one of the families I watched on
TV. I almost expected Alice the maid from "The Brady Bunch"
to appear at any moment to offer us cookies and milk.

I hung out with Gale and his picture-perfect family that day,
but the experience only served to illustrate how different things

were for me at my home, where I'd become the default man of the house.

Because my mom hated to drive, at the age of twelve I began driving her around town when I wasn't in school. I could barely reach the pedals, but Mom had absolute trust in my abilities behind the wheel.

"You're the best driver in town," she'd say. And I believed her.

When I was in eighth grade, my sister Edweena let me borrow her car to take my date, Shannon, to our junior high prom. It wasn't just my driving that impressed her, it was the car: a green '69 Camaro.

That night, Shannon and I were the picture of cool. She was wearing a long flowing dress and I sported a maroon sports jacket, plaid bell-bottom pants, and platform shoes. I remember how I expertly pulled into the school parking lot, with most of our classmates and Mr. Beech, our principal, looking on.

The next morning, Mr. Beech was on the phone to my mother.

"Mrs. Clark, I saw Dwayne drive to school last night."

"Yes?"

"Well, does your son have a driver's license?"

"No, but my Dwayne is an excellent driver."

"But he's not allowed to drive. He's too young. He doesn't have a license," insisted Mr. Beech.

"Well, I said he can drive. I don't know why you're bothering me about this."

And that was that.

Backed up by my mother's confidence in my abilities, I enthusiastically added tasks to my unwritten job description like plumbing, window replacement, and yard work. Mom had finally bought a house. It wasn't new and spiffy, but we were proud. Instead of being renters, we were now homeowners, and at thirteen, I set about the ambitious task of renovating our modest house. I had eyes on turning it into a showplace like Gale's on the hill. I wanted desperately to grab my slice of the American dream—and the sooner the better. I skipped school for weeks to tackle my home improvement project.

First, I wanted to replace a wall in the bedroom. I asked the guy at the lumber store how to do it and it seemed simple enough. That week, a truck pulled up with everything I needed—drywall, mud, tape, and a trowel. I paid for it myself out of my earnings from my job at the recycling center, which I got through a government program for teenagers. I hung the drywall without a hitch and then finished it with new paint.

Then I bought new shag green carpet for the living room, but that job I underestimated. For starters, I couldn't lift the twelve-foot carpet roll once it had been deposited on our front porch. I measured what I would need for the main section of the room and eventually managed to drag the carpet to the front yard, where I had enough room to roll it out and then cut it in half. I got the two pieces into the house, cut them to fit the odd angles of the room, and nailed them into place with carpet tacks.

After that, I took on the backyard, roto-tilling the tough soil and planting what eventually turned into a passable lawn. My mother had no part in any of it. When I started on the bathroom, my mother's contribution was purely aesthetic. "Make it pink," she pronounced. As far as I was concerned, I'd much rather roll out carpet than attend biology class. Life with Mom gave me license to play the part of a man.

My mother, by contrast, didn't take to all aspects of adult responsibility. She struggled with mundane tasks such as paying the bills, made even more stressful by the reality that we seldom had the money to pay them. When bills arrived, she stuffed them in a drawer. Eventually, the calls would start to come in. "Don't let them know I'm here!" my mother would plead.

So I took the calls instead, usually within hours of the lights being turned off or the phone disconnected, "What's the least I can pay?" I asked over and over again. Then I'd dash over to pay the minimum we'd negotiated with whatever cash I could find in the house or get out of my mom. She picked up every extra shift she could and I had my jobs, but without the financial assistance of Edweena, who waited tables, and Linda, who worked part-time at the library while attending college, I don't know how we would have gotten by. Even my older brother, Larry, made it a point to send home a little extra money on occasion.

My mother remained purposefully oblivious. I clearly remember the day I was on the phone negotiating with a bill collector when she pranced happily through the front door, a bag from a local dress shop in each hand. She did not make being the man of the house an easy job.

It might seem as though she was an irresponsible parent, but I like to think that it was her way of including me in her life and preparing me for the future. Whatever her reasons, the unusual responsibilities that I took on made me feel helpful and gave me a tremendous amount of confidence at an early age. What's more, they earned me my mother's gratitude, which was the most important thing in the world to me.

To this day, I believe that the confidence and sense of responsibility she instilled in me as a boy is largely responsible for my success as an adult. There was never any question in my mind that I would be good at what I did because my mother never, ever doubted me. Even though we were poor, Mom always acted as though we were as important and wealthy as movie stars. I understood that we didn't have money to buy every fancy thing we wanted, but I never felt poor. And I never felt neglected. The power of her love and the strength of her belief in me—those two intangibles powered me like jet fuel, keeping me motivated and strong throughout my teen years.

How could I ever doubt myself with that kind of encouragement?

While I was operating as if I was much older at home, at school they still regarded me as a kid. Sometimes a smart-aleck kid. Mr. Segerson, the school wrestling coach, was also my math teacher. In his class, if a kid acted up, it could result in a "hack," which essentially entailed being bent over and hit with a paddle—custom-designed for maximum effect. It seems shocking to talk about it now, an era when we question whether even parents have the right to spank their children, but corporal punishment was alive and well in many corners of America in the 1960s and early 1970s.

It was certainly accepted in Lewiston. One day when I was goofing around with my friend, Mr. Segerson pulled out his hack and requested that I join him in the hall. For the brief moment before the shock of the blow landed on my body, I took in a breath and braced myself. Suddenly I was lifted off the ground and propelled forward. The pain was incredible, knocking the wind out of me and leaving me on the floor, unable to move out of the way even if I had dared to avoid a second blow. Mr. Segerson struck me again and then went back to the classroom. It took me several minutes to collect myself before I could limp into the room and back to my desk. Sitting in my chair was out of the question. I sort of draped myself over my desk for the remainder of the period.

The next day, I would discover the damage to my body: a black and blue bruise that radiated across my backside, almost down to my knees and up towards my kidneys. But that day, the thing that caught my attention was the damage to my brand-new Levi's: a scattering of perforations across the backside, a perfect reflection of the handmade holes drilled in Mr. Segerson's hack.

It didn't take long for my mother to also notice the damage to my jeans. I told her about being hacked and then I showed her my bruised body.

"Goddamn it!" my mother raged. "I'm going to call your teacher and chew his ass out!"

A sense of righteous indignation started to swell up in me as well. This, right here, was why it paid to have a firebrand for a mother. She wasn't going to allow her child to be treated this way. I could see it in her face as she marched to the phone—nobody hits a Clark and gets away with it.

"This is Colleen Clark," I heard her say as I entered the kitchen. "My son Dwayne has just come home and the entire backside of his jeans are ruined."

I could hear Mr. Segerson's muffled voice through the phone, trying to explain what I had done to deserve the hack. My mother and I locked eyes while she listened patiently to his explanation. Then she said firmly, "Mr. Segerson, I don't care if you beat his backside when he deserves it, but you're going to have to pay for his pants. They're his brand-new school pants, and I'm not made out of money!"

It wasn't as bad as being on the business end of a hack, but he got my mother's version of a shellacking. The school paid to replace my jeans. And I took comfort in the fact that I had probably the only mother in town who would stand up to a teacher in that way.

Mother and I became even closer in the months after Granny moved out to live in the nursing home—despite the fact that our conflicting and busy schedules sometimes made it hard to connect.

Before dawn, Mom would rise to get herself ready for a long day, which entailed not only hours working over the stove at the Elks Lodge restaurant but also her two visits to Granny. By the time she returned home she was so exhausted that it was all she could do to get her shoes off and fall into bed. Though I tried to spend quality time with her, most days she was a shadow moving around the house, one that I was vaguely aware of in the pre-dawn hours as I drifted in and out of early-morning dreams. Eventually, I'd pull myself out of bed and get ready to walk to school, go to my classes, and come home in the afternoon. Almost always it was to an empty house.

Most days I'd watch television, but on some afternoons, I rode bikes or played ball with the guys. I had lots of friends, but they came and went with the years. The lonely days made me miss even more how things had been when my brother and sisters were in the house.

Changes were coming though. I was actually growing into manhood—not just acting the part—and experiencing the conflicts and desires of adolescence. At fourteen, I had begun to discover girls, rock and roll, and the torments of peer pressure. My body was beginning to change, too, and the stew of hormones, mixed with a nagging, ever-present feeling of frustration over being without a father, was transforming me into an angry young man.

Still, I loved my mom, desperately, in fact. Most mornings, I woke with a sense of terror that she'd be gone, followed quickly by relief when I realized that she was still here. I knew that, at any time, she could be taken from me and I'd be completely alone. It was my greatest fear.

I'd learned about fear from Mom. She was always afraid. She was frightened by the idea that someone would kidnap her kids, afraid of driving, scared that if we overexerted ourselves we'd drop dead from a heart attack. She was terrified of the dark. Her intense fears were unusual for someone who could be so confident and forceful, but the contrast was just part of who she was.

One Saturday during the summer Mom and I showed up at the nursing home to visit Granny only to be greeted by a concerned nurse standing outside her room. She'd been waiting for us.

"We tried to call," the nurse said. "But you were already on your way."

Mom gasped and gripped my arm for support. "What's happened?"

Granny hadn't been feeling well for some time. It was painful for her to move and she'd been less and less responsive to physical therapy. Mom had worried out loud about this latest turn of events, but she'd also been hopeful that Granny would bounce back. But as the nurse crossed her arms, it became obvious that Granny wasn't getting better, not now or ever.

"Your mother said she's made up her mind. She isn't going to get out of bed anymore," the nurse explained.

"Oh no," Mom whispered.

The nurse nodded. "I'm afraid so. If there's any way you can convince her to change her mind, we really need to get her some exercise on a daily basis."

"I understand," Mom said. "Thank you. I'll talk to her."

The nurse left, walking past us down the hall. Instead of going into Granny's room, Mom led me by the arm, back outside. When we were halfway around the building, she gave me a great hug and started to cry softly. It didn't register with me that the nurse had just delivered a death sentence. Of course, I didn't understand it at the time, but Mom did. Granny was preparing to die.

About eight months later, we received a call at two o'clock in the morning. Granny was in trouble and we should come down right away.

In a flash, Mom and I were in our 1972 Mercury Montego.

"You drive," Mom instructed, even though I was already getting behind the wheel. I sped down the hill so fast over the crest of a small hill that the car actually left the ground like a scene from "Starsky and Hutch." Mom didn't even notice. She just wanted to get there.

Side by side, we ran down the long hallway to Granny's room, but when we got there, it was clear we were too late. Two nurses, both weeping, stood next to her door.

"She passed away about five minutes ago," a nurse said.

Mom fell into the arms of the other nurse and still another came from around the desk to help prop Mom up. All the nurses had come to love Granny's dry British wit and her stories of growing up in the old country.

The women were all sobbing now, and I was left alone in this pocket of abject grief. I wasn't sure what to do or say. I was so numb with shock. I certainly couldn't bring myself to cry, even though I knew I should. It didn't seem real. I peeked into Granny's room and saw her still figure lying on the bed, looking peaceful and asleep but certainly not dead.

After a while, Mom and I went into the room. We held hands, shuffling slowly as we approached her bed, as though we were both afraid to wake her. Granny's skin was ashen. Her lips were parted and her eyes were closed. The room felt charged with energy, but I had difficulty making any sense of it at the time. My heartbeat was in my ears and I couldn't catch my breath, but after a while I calmed down and just looked at her. Mom and I stood in the silence of that room for a very long time.

This was the first time I'd ever seen a person who'd died, and the last time I'd ever see my Granny. It was like being utterly and completely lost, with no hope of rescue. I was sure I'd never recover from the grief.

With the bitterness and spite of a teenager, I selfishly saw this as another example of the cruel joke that my life was becoming, just one more thing that had gone horribly wrong. Granny was dead. Another ally vanished. A piece of my security, the person I'd turned to so many times for advice and love, had been stolen from me. Once again, I felt the sting of abandonment, and I wasn't getting used to it.

Good Days, Bad Days

My sisters and I made another big decision: We decided to move Mom to an Aegis community just ten minutes away from me rather than forty-five. It made little difference to Mom. She was rarely able to track time accurately, generally fluctuating between awareness of immediate needs and long mental absences. To me, though, it was a comfort to know she was just minutes away.

When Mom first moved into assisted living, we had all the best of intentions not to be like those "other families" that visited only on birthdays and holidays. We soon learned that with Alzheimer's, intentions can go astray.

As the months passed, Mom, in fits and starts, began to lose hold of the world around her; there were times when she couldn't even recognize Edweena, and those times were occurring more and more often. It was terrible to watch. For Edweena, the journey was particularly difficult. She would visit Mom regularly, but not as often—not because of the four-hour drive she had to make from Spokane but because she could no longer find ways to bridge the emotional distance that now existed between her and Mom. It was sometimes too painful to even try.

After a family conference, we decided it was time for Mom to move to the facility closest to me. That way, at least one of her children would be available at a moment's notice. We also made the decision to hire a part-time personal attendant. My nephew, Derrick, was now a manager at this new Aegis community, and we were able to hire his wife, Sally, who was then studying nursing, to come for a few hours every afternoon. It was a perfect match on a practical level and it turned out to be a perfect fit emotionally as well. Sally grew to really care for and love my mom.

Within a few days of my mother moving in, Kathy Stewart, the executive director and an exceptional nurse, came to talk with me. She said my mother's behavior reminded her of another case she had worked on. That patient had Parkinson's, another neurodegenerative disease, and it was exacerbating her Alzheimer's symptoms. I knew Parkinson's and Alzheimer's had overlapping symptoms and that it's not uncommon for a patient to suffer from both conditions at the same time. Still, it had never occurred to me that that was the situation for my mom.

We got a second opinion and confirmed Kathy's informal diagnosis. As soon as Mom started her new medications it felt as if the clock had been turned back. Almost immediately, she was transformed. Where she had once required three people to transfer her from her wheelchair to her bed, she was now walking on her own. She was more alert and more energetic. All I could think was: *How did we not see this? And what might her quality of life have been if we had caught this earlier?* Our ill family members depend on us to be their advocates, but it's harder than any of us might think.

Now, we were just grateful. It was wonderful to see Mom and Edweena walk together down the halls again, following the paths in the carpet that help residents find their way, Mom holding onto the handrail cleverly disguised as period wainscoting. Sometimes they even ventured out to the small courtyard to pick tomatoes. She seemed quite at home in this new "hotel." It was if the disease had regressed by two years, giving us some hope and optimism.

Mom started playing Bingo again and working on craft projects. She joined other residents to visit a nearby elementary school where the children read to them; my mom even helped one child sound out several difficult words.

Nonetheless, whether she was having a good day or a bad day, Mom's fear of being alone never seemed to go away. So we tried to compensate. If none of the children were visiting or Derrick or Sally weren't available, the staff made sure she had a nurse or volunteer nearby and Sally made it a point to stop in often. The presence of others helped quite a bit, but if Mom was left alone for even a few moments, she would begin calling, "Are you there? Where are you?" You could sense the panic in her voice. It was as if she was caught between an old self who understood what was happening and a new self who didn't. In that gap lived a swirl of anxiety that couldn't be shaken. She looked, felt, and acted much better, but she still lived in a limbo where her memory and understanding were causing her as much pain as did the loss of those things.

So I visited often, always relieved to see that my mother was one of the first to greet me. She could usually be found sitting next to the concierge desk, chatting with the staff and residents. She greeted visitors and flirted shamelessly with any man she found attractive. She was particularly taken with one of the doctors who made rounds at the facility. "You can come take care of me, honey," she'd inform him with a mischievous grin.

Like many of the residents, Mom made no distinction between her private room and the rest of the building. It was all hers. Sometimes she'd even nap in the lobby; if someone woke her, she didn't hesitate to loudly reprimand: "Shut up! Be quiet! I'm trying to sleep!" Her trademark "colorfulness" had only become more blunt as her filters faded. One day, Mom looked up from her station near the front desk and casually observed of a visitor, "Lady, you have a really big ass."

When I came to visit later that afternoon, Kathy, who had witnessed the outburst, told me the story, all the while trying hard not to laugh out loud.

Of course, Mom had never been shy about giving her opinion. "I don't give a shit what anybody thinks!" was one of her trademark sayings. As she got older, her brusque manner became even more brash and unedited. Long before her decline, I always braced myself whenever we were out at a restaurant, quietly hoping that she wouldn't embarrass us with one of her offhand remarks.

Unfortunately, these lively times with Mom as the veritable hostess of Aegis weren't to last. The progress my mother made when she started taking the Parkinson's medications continued for about six months, then a light seemed to switch again and she reverted back just as dramatically. She stopped getting out of her chair. Her weight dropped. Her ability to focus and recall memories and thoughts regressed to where it had been months before—perhaps even worse.

One day when I came for another visit, Kathy caught me near the front door.

"Hi Dwayne. Colleen had me type a couple of letters for her yesterday. Here, I printed them for you," she said, handing me several sheets of paper.

The letters, to two of her siblings, read:

Dear Peggy,

Hi my darling. I am thinking of you. I hope you are having a Merry Christmas. You are my special sister. I will try to come to see you next year.

Love to you,

Collu

> *To my dearest brother Dennis Callahan,*
>
> *I'll try to come and see you next year. I'm just a poor bugger. I love you darling. I will try to come to see you, my darling, God willing. I hope you get this letter. I'm cracking up over here.*
>
> *Your loving sister,*
>
> *Colleen*

"Pretty cute," Kathy said. "She had a good day yesterday."

I tried to soften the blow. "Peggy and Dennis died many years ago."

"Oh, I'm sorry, Dwayne. I didn't know."

"No, don't worry. How's she doing today?"

"She didn't eat her lunch again."

It had been days since Mom had recognized me. Sometimes I could cultivate an acceptance of who my mother was now—or who she wasn't. I could take her as the person she'd become, gently rubbing her hands, quietly telling her about the weather outside. Sometimes I could sit comfortably watching television with her, as I could with a stranger. And sometimes when I saw her, I felt like a little kid whose mother won't give him what he wants. I wanted her to know me. I wanted my mom back. I missed her.

I prepared myself emotionally once again. As I walked down the short hallway to her room, I heard Benny Goodman playing softly in the public area, and it nearly took my breath away when I recalled how short the time had been since my mom and

I had happily danced to the sounds of the King of Swing in my kitchen. Less than four years. Emotionally, it felt like a lifetime.

As I came into her room, I noticed the scent of the fresh flowers sitting by her bed, and I wondered if she noticed it, too.

"Hi, Mom," I said. "It's me, Dwayne."

My mother had been staring in the direction of the television, but she slowly turned toward me.

"Are those new glasses?" she asked.

"What? Mom, what did you say?"

"I asked if those are new glasses you're wearing," she repeated.

"Yes, Mom, they are," I said, trying to sound casual. "Do you like them?"

My mother looked at my face for a long time. "I do like them," she said, and then turned her gaze back to the television.

These were the cruelest moments—those short-lived breaks when the mom I've always known shows up as if nothing's ever happened.

I tried to keep the joy from rising in me. *It won't last,* I said to myself. Unequivocally. But I couldn't help it. Those few words of recognition made my day.

I had come at lunchtime to help Mom eat, which was more of a pleasure now that she was enjoying her food again. My sister Linda had insisted that we cut Ensure, the dietary supplement, out of Mom's diet, and she had to argue so determinedly with me. (Nutrition supplements are standard procedure when a patient isn't thriving and is losing weight, but they can make some patients feel bloated and actually dampen their appetites.) Still, Linda convinced me we should suspend it for a month, just to see. And she was right. Mom's appetite had bounced back. Her weight held steady. It was a good experiment.

After her fleeting moment of recognition, Mom started staring blankly into space again.

"Mom?"

No response.

"Here you go, Mom. Have a nice drink of cool water."

Dehydration can profoundly affect an Alzheimer's patient's mental state, and Mom more so than most, so I put the cup to her lips and tilted it. A little water spilled down her chin, but I saw her swallow. It took a while, but eventually she drank most of the liquid. Almost immediately, she was making eye contact again. Amazing.

I laid out a small portion of Mom's favorite, not-so-healthy foods—chicken nuggets, French fries, and applesauce—that had just arrived by tray. "Let's have something to eat, Mom," I said, pushing her wheelchair over to the table and sitting next to her. "This looks like great Tasty Food," I encouraged, try-ing to remind her of the "special" foods we'd indulge in when I was growing up. At this point we didn't worry about making healthy food choices, we only worried about getting her to eat anything. Nutrition was more about calories, not a perfectly balanced meal. We just needed to keep her weight up.

The chicken nuggets were all bite-sized, but still, I started cut-ting them in half and putting them into a small pile. Large, com-plicated plates of food overwhelmed her. And since swallowing was difficult, small bites, accompanied by lots of liquids, were essential for her to maintain her interest in eating.

Mom focused on her meal in a way I hadn't seen for a while. She watched me cut the meat. She followed as I brought the fork up to her mouth. But she didn't open her mouth when it arrived. Her eyes caught mine. I didn't see obstinacy, just vague confusion. I touched the chicken lightly to her lips. Her mouth still didn't open. But as I moved the fork away, thinking I'd see if a French fry might prove more enticing, my mother's mouth finally opened. I was observing the slowness and mistiming of her brain, a vivid scientific hypothesis proved in real time. I imagined seeing the invisible neurons and her actions out of sync. Only this was my mother, not a research subject.

"Oh good, Mom," I said. "Would you like some chicken?"

She nodded and I moved the fork back to her mouth, but it had closed again. I could tell by the look of confusion on her face that she had not deliberately closed her mouth.

"Here you go, Mom," I said, trying once more when her mouth opened. Again, her mouth closed as soon as the fork came near. The connections between her brain and her motor control were simply not sharp enough for her mouth to respond when she wanted it to.

I remembered this scenario when my children were babies, just learning how to eat. They, too, would open their mouths well before the spoon arrived and often closed their mouths before the food had been delivered. We made a game of it, coaxing and laughing and spilling more food than they ever ate.

So that's what I did with my mom on this day. Not playing with her like she was a baby, because she was not. For her, the pathways that had just been forming for my children, who were training their mouths to open when their brains commanded it, were now eroding. For my mother, the act of eating had now become a process. Like so many other things, it was no longer automatic. I realized too that I needed to set aside my expecta-tions and bring patience and humor, if I could muster it, to meal times and everything else, just as I did with my children. While it was painful for me to accept, I could only imagine how confusing and frustrating this new reality must have been for my mother.

By the end of lunch, Mom had managed to eat three chicken nuggets, most of the fries, and a couple of spoonfuls of applesauce. It took more than forty-five minutes and she never seemed to recognize me again while I was there. Still, I felt like it was a good visit. I knew that it was dangerous to think of time with my mother that way—a "good visit" or a "bad visit"—but it helped in some odd way. I knew that at some point these moments would cease. This day, though, had been an unexpected gift and I accepted it gratefully.

Angie

After Granny died, I was angry and depressed much of the time, and that simply wasn't who I wanted to be. True, most 15-year-olds aren't who they want to be, but for me, my emotions extended largely from my sense of abandonment. I missed the people who made me feel like I belonged—my father, my brother, my sisters, and my grandmother—and I wanted them back. Would all the people I loved disappear?

These were the larger questions I contemplated, both consciously and unconsciously. At the same time, I had typical teenage thoughts, typical desires. I wanted to be popular. I wanted to be rich. Most of all, I wanted the "normal" Brady Bunch version of the perfect, funny, loving family I'd grown up on. At times, I tried to convince myself that as much as I wanted the American Dream, I wasn't willing to sacrifice my cool, lone-wolf status for it.

In the spring of my sophomore year, I started cutting classes. And I started racing my car. Angie was my first love, a 1966 Midnight Blue Pontiac GTO with a black leather interior and a top speed I regularly pegged at 123 miles per hour. I remember the first moment I laid eyes on her, her blue paint shining in the sun. I agreed to pay my sister's husband $650 for her over the next year, from my current part-time dishwashing job at Cedars Restaurant.

No more afternoons in front of the television for me. From that time on, when I wasn't working, I spent every spare moment under the hood of that car, tuning her up. Once every couple of weeks, I put her on blocks and rotated her tires. I polished her leather seats until they glowed. I propped up two blue pillows, both embroidered with her name, after the Rolling Stones tune that I loved: "Angie."

With no loving in our souls and no money in our coats
You can't say we're satisfied

At first, car racing was about getting girls. But it soon became a passion, a merit all its own. The rush of high speed, the thrill of danger, and the need to compete were like drugs that consumed all my energy and time. I knew I had an edge over the other guys I went up against, thanks to the years I'd spent driving Mom around. And there was something else beyond my experience, a reckless sense of invincibility coupled with a world-weary indifference. I told myself that I just didn't care whether I lived or died, so I was willing to go where others wouldn't.

Sometimes, we raced up the Lewiston "grade," a treacherous spiral of a road, full of switchbacks and hairpin turns. Occasionally, we'd hear about someone getting in a wreck on that road, but it only made it more appealing for the rest of us. We were crazy kids, mad for speed, certain that our youth and daring would keep us safe. In truth, we were very, very lucky.

In quiet moments, when I wasn't smack in the middle of it all, I knew that it couldn't last and that I was wasting precious time. Most of the time, though, I just didn't care. At least, that's what I told myself. It was about living for the moment, a trait my mom had modeled for me all my life.

In the late fall of my sophomore year, I received the wake-up call I needed. It was Friday afternoon, school was out, and I was walking home with my friend Delroy Keller. As we passed the sports fields, Del spotted a powder-puff football game in progress. This was flag football played by girls from our school, mostly cute cheerleaders. The sidelines were packed with adoring moms and dads and boyfriends.

We sat down at the far end of the field, away from the cheering spectators, and watched for a while. The longer I sat there, the angrier I got. Why was I always on the outside looking in? Why didn't I have their rosy-cheeked parents and privileged lives? With the anger swelling up inside me, I told Del that it was time to piss on their powder-puff in a big way.

We did the classic bad-boy maneuver of the time. We bought a dozen eggs at the mini-mart a few blocks away. Del was convinced I'd chicken out, but I showed him. When we got back to the field, I wasted no time. I threw three eggs into the middle of the field where the girls were gathered for a play.

Two eggs splattered harmlessly in the dirt, but the last egg hit one girl in the head. Tina Wonderly screamed bloody murder thinking that it had been a rock and that the runny yolk had been her own blood.

The game stopped and the prank was suddenly out of control. There wasn't any point in running. Randall Pritchard was the first to reach me. He was Tina's boyfriend and a decent guy, who at one time I had played football and baseball with.

"What the hell, Clark?" Randall said, huffing and puffing. He looked at the carton of eggs and then back at me. He pushed me and I held my hands up, palms facing him, indicating I didn't want any trouble. Randall marched forward but hesitated. It could have been all over, but at that moment the hulking, all-state defensive end got to the scene. Suffice it to say, I got my ass kicked and everything else. I thought I was tough, but I didn't know anything. Laid out on the ground, barely conscious, my nose broken and my lip split, I wondered when a parent would come to my aid. But no one did.

Thank God for that. As it turned out, this was my epiphany, the life-changing wake-up call I must have subconsciously wanted. Eventually, I dragged myself to my feet and stumbled the five blocks to our house. Every step felt like a mile. When I made it to our living room, I collapsed on the couch and passed out.

Mom woke me up a couple of hours later. The blood had dried on the couch where my head had landed and I had to peel myself away from the fabric. As I turned to her, she gasped. I tried to tell her I was okay, but my lips were swollen and the blood had dried and cemented them together so it took a moment for me to open my mouth and get the words out.

"Oh my God," Mom said. Her whole body shook as she spoke.

"Mom, I'm fine," I said, trying hard to sound convincing.

"I'm calling the cops!" she blurted.

"No, Mom. Please. You can't call them." I rose from the couch and the room tilted sideways. Every breath, every step was excruciating. Still, I got to her somehow and put my hand over the phone so she couldn't pick it up.

"Please."

She looked me in the eye for a moment. She must have seen my fear and understood that the cops might mean trouble for me. Indeed, there were speeding tickets I hadn't told her about, as well as several final warnings from a pair of officers who knew me on a first-name basis.

Mom wet a dishcloth and helped me back to the couch. She dabbed at my face, but I told her it hurt too much. It was breaking her heart to look at me, and I just couldn't take that on top of everything else, so I slowly got up to go to the bathroom. I snapped on the light and peered in the mirror, and only then did I fully understand and share her horror. As this purple and red monster in the mirror stared back at me and as I heard my mother crying softly in the living room, I made a decision.

In that moment, I understood that anger, pain, and frustration were things that I needed to put away. I never liked the idea of failing in school or getting in trouble. I knew I was better than that, smarter than that. I looked at myself in the mirror and made a promise. This was it. This was the bottom. Now it was time for me to climb up and out and show Mom and everyone else what I was really made of.

I went back into the living room and sat next to my mom and took her hand. "Mom, I need to tell you something," I said. And I told her everything—the partying and the car racing, which she could sort of handle, and the cutting classes and failing grades, too. When I told her that I was flunking out of school, her mouth fell open. I looked right into her eyes. "I'm sorry for this," I said. "I want it to be different. I really do. Can you help me?"

"Oh, Dwayne," she said. "Of course. We'll do whatever it takes."

She hugged me and whispered in my ear, "My son, my son, my son."

For the remainder of the year, I stayed away from my high school in Lewiston. With some help from our church, the following fall I was enrolled in DeSales Catholic High School in Walla Walla, Washington, located about a hundred miles southwest of Lewiston. Even though I had to leave home at sixteen, I knew it was the right choice—the only choice really—and I was determined to make the most of what I knew was a critical opportunity, a second chance.

The plan was for Mom to follow me when she could wrap up the loose ends of our life in Lewiston, chief among them the sale of our house. That fall, as I restarted my sophomore year, I lived with a wonderful couple, Sally and Steve Mele. I'll always be thankful to them for their generous hospitality. Their home was an oasis for me.

It could have been terribly lonely, but having the Meles in my life made the transition exciting and fun. I made friends quickly at DeSales, but I also made it a point to focus on school. Every afternoon, I came home or went to the library to study and I vowed not to race Angie. That was particularly hard to do (I have to confess that I had a few red-light street races), but my desire to win in the classroom and, ultimately, in life largely outweighed my need to prove I had a faster car. This was probably my last chance, and fortunately, by now, I had realized I'd better not screw it up.

I knew I had let down my mom—not to mention myself—and it was time to straighten out and make it right. Mom had toiled too long and too hard for me to fail. I owed her that much—and more.

Lem Visits Mom

Seven months after Mom moved to the Aegis community near my house in Seattle, we came to spend Thanksgiving Day with her. She didn't know it was Thanksgiving, but she seemed to enjoy it, especially her conversation with my best friend, Lem, who had joined us for dinner. A big man at 6 feet 2 inches tall and 270 pounds, Lem is one of the most caring, jolly, soulful people I know. For me, he's long been the one friend that I can talk to about anything and everything at any time.

Lem asked me about Mom's condition when we stepped away momentarily from the gathering. "It's funny," I answered, "she can remember certain things from long ago, but not what she had for breakfast or that today is Thanksgiving."

He asked what I meant, so I agreed to show him. We sat down with Mom and started to chat. "Mom, I told Lem you fought in the war against the Japanese during World War II."

"Yes that's right," she recalled. "I wore a… I wore… the thing on my head." She struggled to find just the right word. "Um, why can't I think of it? Oh, yes, I wore a tam, the little beret that was part of my uniform."

Mom was obviously proud of her service. "I was the Morse Code instructor!"

"Really?" Lem said, engaged and impressed with my mother.

"Yes! I taught new operators and I had to tell people when an attack would occur," she explained.

"So Mom," I interjected, "if I wanted to say, 'The Japanese are coming,' how would you say that in Morse code?" She thought about it for no longer than ten seconds and then began making tones that mimicked that of a telegraph machine. Di dit di dit dot dot, dit dit dit, dot dot dot dit. (The actual, Morse code translation is: - .... / .--- .- .--. .- -. . .... / .- .-. . / -.-. --- -- .. -. --. .-.-.-)

As she spit out the code sequences with amazing accuracy, I could see her tapping or counting on her fingers just as she had been trained to do more than fifty years before.

"Wow!" Lem exclaimed. "That is impressive!" We gave Mom about three more phrases to figure out. By this time I went online to track what she was saying with the Morse code translation. She'd nailed it every time.

Her short-term memory was almost gone—I would have never asked her who the current U.S. president was—but her long-term memory was being used more than ever before and it was amazingly clear and concise.

Four years later, Lem asked to go with me on another visit to my mom. He knew from our conversations that she was nearing death, and this was his generous way of supporting me and sharing her memory.

I think he was expecting to see a woman who was very sick physically but still able to interact with us. What he got was just the opposite. "Her skin is beautiful, she looks so peaceful. But she isn't communicative at all," he said.

Mom slept through the entire visit, not uttering a single word. "This is hard," Lem said. "I don't know really what to say."

Indeed, it is awkward visiting someone who says nothing and sleeps in front of you. So I comforted Lem by sharing my own coping skills. "I just try to do what I think she would want.

Make sure she is clean, warm her hands with mine, and make sure she has her hair done and make-up on. That is so important to Mom."

Lem and I both held Mom's hands and told stories. He told her things about me that she might like to hear. We talked about the influence that each of our mothers had on us. We joked about all the crazy things they did that somehow made their way into our DNA. Then I gave Mom a kiss and told her, "I love you." Her eyes popped open and she said, "I love you."

Lem looked at me in amazement. "Wow," he commented. "What a wonderful phrase to remember when you don't remember any more."

Part 4.

Being in the Now:
This Is Our Life

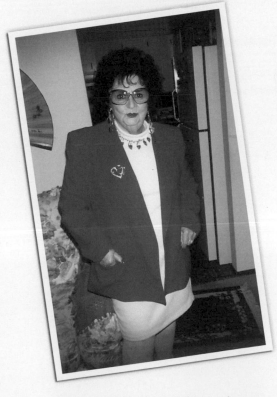

Post Falls, Idaho 1998: Colleen at Christmas

The rest of the night was filled with mom, telling crazy and inappropriate stories, punctuated with more hysterical laughter. Mom was as high as a kite and my buddies were right along with her for the ride. Forty years later when I admitted to mom what happened, she refused to believe that we got her high. She also denied what happened.

On grade 1978, st on an the ked name, crewd the f my her della un She I'd mer For one th After th

Dwayne and Colleen at DeSales High School graduation in Walla Walla, Washington 1978

HOW MUCH IS ENOUGH?

I came across a poem in 2007 by an unknown author, and after reading and re-reading it, I wanted to share it with every family, every person, who ever shared the struggle with Alzheimer's disease. To me, it was, and remains, such a vivid reminder of the ways we're asked to let go and, at the same time, hold on for dear life.

> *I need you*
> *To not ask me to remember,*
> *To not try to make me understand,*
> *Let me rest and know you're with me,*
> *Kiss my cheek and hold my hand.*
>
> *I'm confused beyond your concept,*
> *I am sad and sick and lost,*
> *All I know is that I need you*
> *To be with me at all cost.*
>
> *Do not lose your patience with me,*
> *Do not scold or curse or cry,*
> *I can't help the way I'm acting,*
> *Can't be different, though I try.*
>
> *Just remember that I need you,*
> *That the best of me is gone.*
> *Please don't fail to stand beside me!*
> *Love me 'til my life is done.*

The poem rang so true and so deep to me as it reminded me of how close I was to my mother my whole life—even during the stretches when I didn't spend that much time with her. After moving out and going to college, I probably talked with her three times a week by phone, which was unusual compared to many young adults sowing their wild oats and establishing themselves in their work and relationships. She was always the one I would call when something special occurred in my life, and she always visited me once or twice a year wherever I was living and working. She'd stay a week—just enough time to reignite our memories and have some fun, but not so long that we would get on each other's nerves.

For at least twenty-five years this was our relationship. When Mom moved into assisted living, I made it a priority to see her four or five times a week the first few months. I wasn't going to be one of those bad family members who dumps Mom off and never comes back to visit. In my disdain, it was easy to make all kinds of judgments about "those" people. But after a few months, four to five visits a week dwindled to three visits a month. While I made sure she would see someone in the family multiple times a week, and we'd bring her to our house for visits, that didn't change the fact that I was seeing her a lot less.

I rationalized it to friends and colleagues with details about my busy schedule or explanations of why it was logistically impossible to see her four times a week, but those were excuses. Excuses I shared often with so many others, even myself. I wondered: *If I see Mom twenty days a year, is this enough to be deemed a "good" son?* That's more than I used to see her after I grew up and left home. But I still wondered: *Should I be there more?* My mom visited my grandmother two times a day, every day, when she was in the nursing home. Was that the measure of being a good child? I started to be less judgmental about those family members who chose not to visit so often.

As CEO of Aegis, I knew that it was important to me and my family to make a commitment of time at the beginning, but it wasn't a commitment we were always able to keep as we balanced the important responsibilities of our own lives, our own future. *How many hours, how many days, how many years should we spend on a life that is passing versus the life that is ahead of us?* It was a question I pondered often.

There were new challenges to deal with at each stage of Mom's illness. In the beginning her cognitive awareness was very much intact. She'd long to be with people and she'd plead with us not to leave. We needed a strategy—excuses really—to leave, saying we were running to the store or needed to get something from the car. It was heart-wrenching, of course. Before we arrived for a visit we'd worry about how we were going to part. No matter how happy the visit, we would leave in so much pain. If the visit caused so much agitation, it was easy to begin creating the justification: *Maybe it's better if I don't go, if I don't put everyone through the trauma.*

Ironically, as the Alzheimer's got worse, the visits got easier. The forgetfulness took away the stress. There was vulnerability and a need and a quietness that pulled us in. In the very late stages, it was hard to see any value at all in going. My mom, like most Alzheimer's patients, was not talking and mostly sleeping. But I knew that our presence was healing. Touching, speaking, and comforting all provide dignity and love—no matter what age or condition someone is in.

Facing Alzheimer's is scary and odd and disappointing. All of our childhood wishes are right there with us as grown men and women of forty, fifty, or even sixty years old. We do what we can, and maybe a little more than we can, but it feels like so little and like it can never be enough. If your parent is alive today, hug them. Look them in the eye and tell them they did a great job. I don't care if you believe it or not. Look at them, study their smile, listen to their laugh, feel their touch. Watch the manner in which they walk and eat their food, and even if it is bad tell them it is good. Give them the respect of listening to their same story for the one-hundredth time and laughing at it.

Our parents, like us one day, have finite time. As I continued my visits, I watched my mother and could only cling to memories of her smile, her laugh, her jokes, her mannerisms. She was gone, not physically, but in terms of the person I had known my whole life. She looked through me as if I was a ghost. I tried to close my eyes and think of her as she was, as she would want me to think of her—but I struggled to get past her current condition.

Waiting for Her to Return

Mom's Alzheimer's had progressed substantially. Visiting her now was a different experience and it was easy to doubt the value of being there. Today when I arrived, she was in her wheelchair with the TV on, but once again she was mentally somewhere else. I sat down next to her, waiting for a sign of her awareness to return. As usual I had come at mealtime, as I could at least try and feed her and feel a sense of purpose. This time, I was able to get her to take a few bites of chicken, and eventually she ate the carrot cake as well. As the night wore on, though, Mom receded further and further into her own world until she was totally removed from reality, half in and half out of consciousness. I put on my coat and prepared to leave.

"I'm afraid to die," Mom peeped in a little girl's voice. "I don't want to die, but I'm not going to be around much longer, I think."

I took her hand, leaned down, and kissed her forehead.

"Try not to worry about that now," I said.

"I can't help it," she said and rolled away from me.

Mom had always been afraid of death. Since I was a young boy, she had talked about it, and in the past thirty years the fear had intensified to an almost absurd level. Her Catholic faith had never served her against this fear even though she had prayed to God all her life, asked for intercession from the saints, and talked about heaven. I often wondered how firm her faith was. In some ways, I sensed that she never really believed in heaven but prayed just in case it was true, just to cover her bases. I wondered if Mom's fear of death at times shaped her faith, if she believed that, at some level, she could negotiate her fate. She used to ask me to pray for her to live longer and if she had unexpected pains or aches she would warn us that she was afraid and might be dying at that moment.

It seemed like such a waste to me. Why not think you are going to live fifty years longer even when you are ninety? To me, there is no risk in that philosophy. If you die at ninety, plus one day, you have squeezed all the juice out of life and not wasted one second worrying about your fate. When you die, you die. It's inevitable and natural.

At least that's how I've tried to think of death in the past, no doubt as a counter-measure to Mom's fears of it. But as I put a hand on Mom's shoulder and said goodbye, I was suddenly gripped by the fear that this would, indeed, be the last time I saw her, that I would be alone in the world, that I would be lost. It was the fear of my youth, and though it didn't last very long, it left me feeling heavy and sullen.

The final stages of Alzheimer's are, by far, the most painful to witness. The body shuts down completely and the afflicted is reduced to a warm body, lying in a bed, barely able to swallow.

I wished Mom peace. I didn't want her to suffer. I knew how much her continued decline would scare her. I was terrified that, at the end of this, all she would have were her fears. If my presence could bring her a little peace, it would make this last transition a little easier to bear. It was about her now, not me.

On my way to the main area, I passed a resident sitting at a beautiful oak desk, carefully typing on an old-fashioned type-writer. He might have been filling out a service order, or composing a legal argument, or writing a novel. It didn't matter.

What struck me was his purposefulness, which I sensed gave him comfort and meaning.

I recognized the gentleman. When I was walking by his room once, I had noticed a handwritten note along with the other mementos displayed in the memory box that hung outside his door. When he saw me looking at the letter, the gentleman invited me into his room to chat and explained that he had been an obstetrician. The note was a thank-you letter from the parents of the first baby he had helped deliver.

He was not alone in this activity. The memory boxes are made available to help everyone in the community. Each resident or their family members fill the boxes with important objects as visual cues to help the person find their room. The boxes also remind us that there is so much more than we can see of the person in front of us now. The person is not their disease. They may not be able to feed or dress themselves without assistance, but they are not children.

Most have lived long lives, punctuated with rich stories. Amazing stories like that of my mother—the girl Collu who rode elephants to school in India, enlisted in World War II, and selflessly (most of the time), hilariously, whole-heartedly raised four children on her own in a little American mill town. My mother had sweated and struggled for me; supplemented our underfunded grocery budget with "leftovers" from her restaurant jobs, and insisted my prospects were just as good as the Kennedys'. And now that I had made good on her dreams for me, she sometimes didn't even know who I was. Now that I could give her diamonds and fur coats, all she wanted was for me to hold her hands because they chill easily. And even though I was becoming a stranger to her, I had warm hands.

OUR HOUSE

Leaving Lewiston for Walla Walla meant that I was away from home and on my own for the first time, so I visited my mother almost every weekend. It made it harder to adjust to life in Walla Walla, as I would blow out of town right after school every Friday, but seeing Mom always made the drive worthwhile. We would take up right where we left off. My sisters would come by and we all ate dinner together. That family bonding fortified me for another week back at school.

After three months, Mom cemented her plans to move to Walla Walla to be with me. The day she pulled into town she went straight to a job interview. There was an opening for a full-time cook at the Elks Lodge in Walla Walla, so within hours of arriving, she had landed the job. When we finally saw each other that day, we were both excited and hopeful, but my optimism about starting a "new life" with Mom would be relatively short-lived.

We found an apartment, but it was located in a no-man's land of parking strips and empty lots. The small side yard was difficult to distinguish from the parking lot as both were choked with weeds.

For our first meal together, we had to use lit candles because the power hadn't been turned on. I told Mom about school and my new "A" average and she sang my praises: "There's no question about it. Now that you're away from that criminal element, there's only one way for you to go." She pointed her finger to the sky. "All the way up."

After dinner, we unloaded the last of the boxes from her car. I quickly noticed that items were missing, most notably the TV. I asked her about it and she led me inside and sat me down. After batting her eyes and breathing deeply, as if she were preparing to hold her breath underwater, she took both of my hands in hers.

"My son," she said, "I lost the house."

I held her stare and waited for the punch line.

"I didn't pay the taxes and the county took it back."

I just blinked at her and waited for her to continue. *She can't be serious,* I thought.

"I just forgot. I got busy and forgot."

My mouth fell open, but I still held out hope. There was nothing Mom liked better than a good "I gotcha!"

But then she looked down at her hands and began to tug at her fingers.

"I just lost track of the taxes. I mean, you're the one who usually takes care of these things. Without you to help, I wasn't sure what to do."

"Jesus Christ, Mom!" I shot back. "I'm 16 years old—I'm the one who's supposed to be a kid here!"

I calmed down and asked, "How did it happen? I don't understand." Inside, I was clinging to that last shred of hope that maybe, just maybe she was joking. The house was our family's one and only asset. I couldn't process how this could have happened. I accepted that Mom was flighty, but this was beyond irresponsible.

"I really don't know how it happened," she tried to explain. "It's like I told you. I don't understand how this whole tax thing works. I just don't get it all."

"So, you just never bothered to figure it out?" I accused her. I was still trying to understand how things could have gotten to this point.

Mom sighed and ran her fingers through her hair.

"Yes, my son. Now don't beat me up over this. Let it go. It's over. I borrowed some money from your brother and sisters. And I've got this job now so we'll be fine. But I had to sell a lot of our stuff."

"You sold the TV, didn't you?" I said, voicing my worst fear.

"I did," she replied. "I had to."

I breathed a long sigh and looked around our new home. Near the ceiling in the corner, there was a little patch of green mold that seemed to glow florescent in the half-light.

I was slowly filling up with a new sense of dread, but I didn't let Mom see it. I understood that we had to stay together on this, that laying blame would push her.

"Well," I said. "We needed a new TV anyway."

She laughed out loud, relieved, and gently slapped the table with her open palm.

"Oh, my son, I knew you'd find the joke in this. It's not the end of the world. It will just be like camping for a while. That's all."

I nodded and smiled and continued to play it off as though it wasn't a big deal, as she predicted the coming day when we'd laugh over it, the day when I was president of the United States or a senator or a great lawyer. And I agreed with everything she said. I pretended that everything was okay and that everything would be great.

In reality, of course, I was shattered that she'd lost the house, furious that I no longer had a television. Although I'd pretty much let Mom off the hook for her mistake, I was especially bitter that we'd lost the only thing we really owned. The house was more than a financial loss, it was part of our history.

That night, lying there in the dark with blankets and the hard floor underneath me, I renewed my promise that I would be everything my mom dreamed I could be. President. Senator. Lawyer. I wouldn't let my mind go to that dark place: That fantasy place where everything would have been different, better, if I had had a father who took care of me, who thought I mattered, who showed up at Little League games to root for me as I minded third base. I would see myself in a different light, a young man with his own purpose in life, someone who made a difference in the lives of others, and most important, a man who would never, ever leave his children to ask questions with unknowable answers while they lay on a cold, hard floor for a bed.

"My mom believes in me," I told myself. That was what mattered. Not the losses and things I didn't have.

My mom believes in me.

I felt a warmth building in me as I repeated my mantra and thoughts of my dad slowly dissolved.

My mom believes in me.

It was all I needed. There was no sense in holding on to the things I couldn't change. It would always be there. It would always make me sad. But I wouldn't let it stop me or change me. It would make me stronger somehow.

My mom believes in me. My mom believes in me.

I repeated the phrase over and over until I finally fell sleep.

So many years later, I still remembered that night and the moment when I finally let go of the things I couldn't have and fully embraced the relationship that was the most important in my life.

Only now do I understand what that night really meant: After so many years of my mom believing in me, I was finally learning to believe in myself.

Walla Walla 1976
Potato Soup

A week into our life in Walla Walla, Mom sat me down again, performing her anxious ritual of touching her face and primping her hair before she could speak. I waited nervously as she breathed her deep breaths. What could it be this time? We had no house to lose.

Finally, she took her purse, set it on the table between us, and took out a five-dollar bill. She placed it on the table between us and stared at it as though she expected the money to turn into a butterfly and flutter away.

"I don't get it," I said. "Five bucks?"

"That's all we have," she said.

"No way," I whispered. "How?"

"First and last month's rent. The new accounts for the phone and the utilities and the groceries I bought last week. Gas for the car."

"Five bucks," I sighed.

"Stop saying that," she ordered and took the bill from the table and put it back into her purse.

"I don't get paid for another ten days," she said. "And I can't ask them for an advance when I've just barely started working there."

"What are we going to do?" I asked.

"I don't know. We'll think of something," she said.

This was not good—even by Mom's shaky standards. We never had much money, but this was the only time I recall having essentially *no* money at all. I was stunned by the news and couldn't figure a way out. I suppose we could have gone back to my brother or my sisters, but there was the issue of Mom not wanting to tell any of them why she needed it: pride. Even at her lowest, she was an intensely proud woman.

Once again, it was just me and Mom. We had to rely on each other, and I knew we'd find a way. We always did, I told myself, at the same time silently willing twenty bucks to fall from the sky.

We spent those last five dollars on more groceries, but within a few days, those were gone as well. We had to survive another week before Mom would get her paycheck from the Elks Lodge restaurant. Though we had done the math and knew the food wouldn't last, we were still surprised to find our cupboards and refrigerator completely void. When you get to the point of actually having no food, and you've always had food before, it just doesn't compute.

Fortunately, Mom had a plan.

Looking back, her decision that day made perfect sense. And I'm still grateful because it turned out to be one of the single most important turning points in my life, a lesson learned that I will always carry with me.

The plan was simple. Mom would steal some food—"borrow" in her words—from the Elks' kitchen, to get us through the week. She'd go in before dawn and grab some potatoes, the least expensive item from the Elks' inventory. I would wait outside in the getaway car.

Upon hearing her scheme, I lobbied for some steaks or prime rib, as well. Mom snapped back and quickly set the record straight. "We don't steal, Dwayne! This is a one-time thing. We'll replace every single potato and then some. And we'll pay them back with interest as soon as I get my paycheck."

It was settled then. Mom was supposed to start her shift at the Elks' restaurant to prep food at 6 a.m., but instead, I drove her to work two hours early. I pulled around to the back alley, dropped Mom, kept the car running, and waited. Before too long she re-emerged from the back door with a bucket full of potatoes. She handed them off to me without a word, but the look in her eyes reaffirmed everything I already knew. She was Bonnie and I was Clyde. Together, we'd make it through whatever the world threw at us. We were determined and we weren't going to let a little thing like no money and no food stop us. She strode back to the door and it slammed as she went back inside. I sped away down the alley as the sky turned orange. The day was just beginning.

That night, Mom and I made potato soup. We peeled the potatoes and cut them into cubes. Then we boiled them until they were soft and mashed them up, adding the last of the milk and butter we had left, along with half a Walla Walla sweet onion and some salt and pepper. We were both hungry in a way we'd never been before.

That first night the soup was delicious, as good as anything I've ever had. After we'd finished, I listed off ingredients that would make the soup even better: carrots, mushrooms, garlic, peppers. "That's going to have to wait until I get paid," Mom insisted, again emphasizing that our caper would never be repeated.

At some level, we'd always taken food for granted. But now, with this being the only thing to eat in our little house, it took on a special meaning that remains with me today. I think about that one meal almost every time I sit down at the dinner table, never taking for granted just how lucky I am to be eating anything, much less a nourishing hot meal. It was a lesson that would shape my life and influence my future in ways I couldn't even imagine then.

We ate that soup all week long. It was cold enough outside that we could store the soup pot in our milk box, which sat outside, right next to the front door. We heated it on the gas stove—which, thankfully, hadn't been turned off. But on the third day, the power was disconnected so we ate by candlelight and talked into the night.

"You have to make me a promise, my son."

"What?" I said, slurping my soup.

"Don't ever forget where you came from. No kidding. Don't forget this," she said, holding a spoonful of soup between us. "This is very important to remember. Always remember."

"Okay," I said, still more interested in eating than hearing advice.

Mom paused dramatically and waited until she got my full attention. Then she drove her point home:

"If you ever have people working for you, treat them like family, support them, and help them when they need it because things don't always work out for people. They probably won't ask you for help or tell you their troubles, but you can tell when things aren't right for people if you just pay attention to them. Be there for your people and they will always be there for you."

Mom's message sunk in—it would later become a foundational philosophy when I started Aegis Living—and we did survive. We lived on potato soup for a week and we didn't starve. Mom had lunch at the Elks Lodge and I charmed some of the girls at school into sharing lunch with me. It wasn't easy and it wasn't fun. But we never told anyone that our refrigerator was empty. We just got by.

And when Mom's first paycheck finally arrived, we got the power turned on and went on a grocery run. Most importantly to Mom, we bought a bag of potatoes and she returned them to her employer; in fact, she returned more potatoes than she had "borrowed." As she had promised, we paid the loan back with interest.

After things leveled off, life was good in Walla Walla. We even got a new TV. DeSales High School was a great place to go to school, a calm environment, far from the trouble I'd made before. Beyond my own expectations (but not Mom's), I actually made the dean's list with a 3.87 grade point average in my sophomore year, nearly a straight "A" student.

All in all, I learned an extremely valuable lesson: Good people can go through the hardest of times. I knew now to watch for signs that people may need help, to recognize those signs, and to be kind, not judgmental. I would never forget that people sometimes do desperate things when they find themselves in desperate situations.

April Fools'—Loss Buried in Such Small Things

Despite her experiences growing up as a privileged daughter of a British railroad man in India, my mother had spent her adult life as an immigrant in America. She had certain cultured airs that reflected her childhood but she also displayed a cultural naiveté that was not uncommon to the immigrant story, leaving her always a little bit behind her peers and a tad middle-brow. The two markedly different experiences that informed her outlook left her with a desperate need to learn—and try to inhabit—all that was great about America, her adopted country. Or at least fantasize that she and her children could be part of it.

As a result, she was gullible in weird ways. She actually read the *National Enquirer* and *Star* magazine, believing in some strange way that the pages could somehow make her a better American. Worse, she believed that long-since-dead Elvis was alive and well and hanging out on an island in the Pacific. The wilder the story, the more quickly she embraced it as fact.

For us, Mom was an easy mark for our outlandish pranks. They soon evolved into a family tradition, highlighted by our annual, over-the-top April Fools' jokes. My brother and sisters were quite creative at coming up with great ideas, and having gotten an early start, I was quite good at "getting her" as well. With her easy laugh and sense of fun, Mom was the perfect victim, and our success was aided by the fact that even after twenty years of pranking her, she always seemed to forget that April 1 was April Fools' Day.

As an adult, I would take days and weeks contemplating and debating new prank ideas until I came up with something truly over the top. The key to making it work was, like the *National Enquirer*, I always made sure there was that element of plausibility to the story.

When I was living in Virginia, for example, I called her and announced: "I've sold everything."

"What do you mean you sold everything?" she asked me, startled and worried. She knew how hard I'd been working and how ambitious I was.

"I've sold everything." I repeated. "All my worldly possessions. All the kids' possessions. I've decided to move to a commune in Oregon. I realize how misguided I've been and we're just going to live a very simple life and wear simple saffron robes and shave our heads."

She begged me to reconsider, totally caught up in the idea that I would completely change my life and everything she knew about me.

Once I shouted "April Fools!" she laughed, with the same intensity that she had worried only moments before. Our "deal" was still on—you and me together, surviving and conquering the world.

Another time I called and told her I had some really big, exciting news to share and she better sit down because it was really hard to believe. I explained that my fifty-year-old sister Linda was pregnant with twins. For a second, I thought the shock was going to kill her.

Then there was the time I completely played to her fantasy of getting rich and "making it." In my most serious voice I called her on April 1, first thing in the morning, and explained that I'd won the Powerball lottery—to the tune of $300 million. I told her I wanted to take her to Olympia to receive the check. She was giddy and overwhelmed with excitement and I already felt bad for the letdown that was to come, even though I was enjoying every second of the joke. She was talking a mile a minute. "Oh my God, what should I wear?" she asked. "We're going to be on TV. Can I wear a hat? What do you want me to say to the press?"

Like all the times before, I gently said, "Hey, Mom, April Fools." And in true mom form, she yelled, "God damn it, you got me again. Why are you such an ass?" And then she'd laughed her head off.

It was one of our favorite days of the year. April Fools' became a "two-fer"—a challenge and pleasure for me and a joy for her. For more than twenty years, I'd set her up, and each joke would be more hilarious than the previous one. As small an occasion as it was, it became a tradition as strong as any birthday or holiday celebration.

Sadly, as Mom declined, I would decline as well. I couldn't have predicted that. Her loss of understanding and enjoyment meant the loss of things that held special meaning for me and made me feel good about myself and our special way of relating. Like the April Fools' tradition.

It happened gradually, but at some point April 1 came and went for us without any jokes, without any laughter. Mom didn't "get it" anymore. The fun was gone and it didn't make sense to plan another "Can You Top This?" scenario. It's such a routine day that most people let it go by unnoticed, but for me, an uncelebrated April Fools' Day was tantamount to genuine loss. Alzheimer's stole that connection and the way it made me see myself—from me as well as from her.

We are defined and bound by our relationships. If we lost all our friends today, all our family members and co-workers, we would become untethered, our foundation dropped out from under us. Who would we be? When our lives are caught up with a key person who has a disease like Alzheimer's, all our attention goes to that person and how we can help and make them better. It's only over time, when the changes are so great, that we realize our focus on the other person's losses has concealed the fact that we are also losing parts of ourselves.

We can try to bury those rituals and traditions, whether it's Mother's Day, Mom's birthday, or April Fools' Day. We can focus on getting through day by day. We can go for long periods of time ignoring the changes and avoiding making plans because we never know what's next beyond making the person comfortable today. But it's those memories, those rituals, those experiences that form the relationships we had and identify the person we are in the world.

Sometimes we cling harder to those special times or they take on new and unanticipated importance. It's our way of dealing with *our* needs, not just the needs of our loved one—and, as I would realize, that is just as necessary.

HEARTACHE

When Mom suffered her heart attack in the restaurant in 2000, doctors put in an artificial pacemaker to regulate her heartbeats. Now the battery powering that medical device was failing and we had to make a very difficult decision about whether or not to put Mom through the surgery to replace it.

I spoke to her cardiac surgeon, who explained that the procedure itself was quite safe, but that surgery itself and the potential for infection did pose risks. Still, the decision was even bigger than that. It was a huge ethical issue for our family. Should we put our eighty-six-year-old mother through the pain and trauma of surgery and recovery? Did we have the right to decide for her? Or should we let the pacemaker battery die and accept the natural course of what would follow?

By keeping her heart beating, we would be potentially adding years to her life. But given the cruel evolution of Alzheimer's and what it does to a person's body in the late stages, would that be a good thing or a bad thing? Even the cardiologist asked me, "Wouldn't it be kinder if your mother just went to sleep as opposed to being slowly destroyed by the effects of Alzheimer's?"

I wasn't sure how a son was supposed to answer this question. This was a very painful decision our family had to face together. My sisters agonized over it, and I was confused and sad, absolutely in shock that I would have to help make a decision like this for my mother. I second-guessed my thinking constantly.

I wanted to do what was right, but I wasn't sure anymore what that was.

Eventually, my sisters and I met and decided we were going ahead with the surgery, as it really was what my mother would have wanted. She always instructed us: "Keep me alive at any cost." The day of the operation, we had to arrive very early in the morning. Though 4:50 a.m. seems early to put on a suit and tie, that's what I did. I'm not sure why I felt the need for formality, but I think it was out of respect for my mother. As was always the case whenever I saw her now, I didn't know if this would be my last time with her. I wanted to be prepared and appropriate, whatever that meant.

We had coordinated a "cabulance" to transport her to the hospital, and I timed it so I would arrive at the same time she did. As I pulled into the nearly empty parking lot, however, a big fire truck and aide car pulled in front of me. This delay and their extra-slow driving irritated me greatly. I wanted to get into the hospital and be with my mom.

As soon as I could, I pushed by and raced to the top floor of the garage to park. As I arrived to meet my sisters, I noticed a group of firemen wheeling my mom in. The cabulance had forgotten to pick her up, and the rescue squad, who I was so upset with just minutes earlier, had transported my mom instead. I felt like an idiot. They had been so careful with her and accommodating.

Inside, we explained to the surgery nurse that Mom had Alzheimer's and could not really communicate for herself. Over the last few months Mom had progressed in her Alzheimer's stages and could no longer connect enough words to create full sentences. All she could do was pull forth a word or two at a time, a fact that was frustrating for her, as well as everyone around her.

Mom was obviously confused and scared, so my sisters and I did our best to reassure her and calm her down. The nurse was very kind as she poked Mom's arm to find a vein and start the IV. As with many seniors, though, Mom's veins were small and prone to collapsing. After enduring a few unsuccessful attempts, Mom let out a yelp and made the clearest statement I'd heard her make in three years. "Take that goddamn thing out or I will slap your face!" *Wow, now that's my old mom,* I thought.

Even as I tried to calm my mother down, I turned to my sister in disbelief. "Did she just say what I think she said?" The fact that Mom realized she had just had pain in a specific area was remarkable. The fact that she could fully articulate it was epic.

The surgery lasted a little over an hour, and all went well. The staff was exceptional, and the hospital CEO even came down and spent time with us. Mom came out of anesthesia without incident and was wheeled to her hospital room. I stayed with her, and surprisingly, she continued to speak in long sentences throughout the day. At one point, when a nurse took her blood pressure. Mom turned to me and stated, "This thing is much too tight—can you take it off my arm?"

Given the circumstances, it was amazing how relatively normal she appeared to be. When she recovered enough to return to her Aegis home, the executive director, who is also a nurse, remarked that it was as if Mom had gone back to where she was a year ago. I was intrigued by this seeming advance and immediately started calling researchers and physicians that I knew to ask what might have caused it. Most believed that the new pacemaker increased her blood flow, enabling her brain to get more oxygen, which improved verbal capacity. Another theory emerged that because the body often responds to pain by shooting adrenaline into the bloodstream, they may have jumped over Mom's blocked neurological receptors, enabling her mind to transmit information again. Our University of Washington longevity specialist was so impressed that she said it was going to be the topic for her research team that day.

We couldn't know if Mom's resurgence would last a day or a year, but I was happy to have her spark back—no matter how long it stayed. She was telling us we did the right thing by her.

Unfortunately, although her physical recovery from the surgery continued to go very well, her mental capacity regressed back to her previous condition over the next two months. In short order, Mom was a frail facsimile of her past self, and I feared that she was living the last months of her life. We all wondered about the end but no one knew exactly how it would manifest.

When I heard that she was slipping back to her deteriorated state, I couldn't bring myself to go and visit her. One, two, three, four, and finally seven weeks passed before I worked up the courage to go and see her. My daughter, Ashley, went with me as a motivator to make sure I completed the visit. We brought Mom her favorite high-calorie treats to entice her to eat.

When we entered the Aegis community, I put on my happy face as staff greeted me. Mom looked good, her hair done and makeup on. She was sitting in the lobby, her eyes closed, listening to entertainment.

We wheeled her off to the activities room to have some quiet time. Ashley said, "Gram, we brought you some carrot cake, yours and Dad's favorite." It was an attempt to spark a memory: My mother had brought me carrot cake for my high school graduation, even though I hate carrot cake. When I told her, "Mom, you know I hate carrot cake," she responded, "Yes, but I love it!"

To our delight, she gobbled up the carrot cake and, when my feeding was not fast enough, she pulled off chunks of the cream cheese frosting and popped them in her mouth. However, when we tried to carry on a conversation, Mom just stared at us, though by the look on her face, she appeared to be trying to locate the file that matched our faces to the memory. We asked her questions, hoping, praying, for some type of response. The best we got was a shake of the head and an "uh ha."

When she got to a piece of carrot or a nut that she didn't like, she would spit it out on the floor, like a farmer would a wad of chewing tobacco. This was so not the mother I knew, an English woman with a proud background; good manners were always so important to her. The disease, though, manages to strip away any acquired values, pretenses, and political correctness from its victims. Alzheimer's patients display a pureness, an innocence as they are rendered back to what they are at their core, not who they are raised up to be, who they are supposed to be.

My daughter and I talked and tried to make Mom laugh, a simple thing, it would seem, but it was the simple things that I yearned for now that I didn't have them anymore. My daughter had gotten engaged two weeks before, and she said to me, "Dad, the one thing that I am most sad about is that I couldn't call and share the moment with Gram." Those words shot through me, so painful that I nearly cried. As I fought back my emotions, I realized how much this disease steals from people, the essence of life and joy.

Mom polished off her carrot cake and some of the other desserts. We wheeled her in for dinner. As we were leaving, I bent down and kissed her and stated: "I love you."

"I love you," she said, clear as day. There were some things this disease couldn't steal.

LEAVING THE NEST

In the fall of my senior year of high school, I established a relationship with a friendly guidance counselor and told her that I wanted to go to college. She explained that through the network of Catholic schools that included DeSales I could gain entry into an accredited four-year program at Chaminade University, thanks, in part, to my grades, participation in sports, and student leadership. There was only one problem: Chaminade was in Honolulu, Hawaii.

The day I broke the news to Mom, she put her hands on my shoulders and shook me lightly. "My son, that's so far away. There would be an entire ocean between us. It's too far, I think."

I didn't have an answer. Sure, I could have gone to Washington State University, which was nearby, or even a community college, so that we could still live together. And I considered this. But I needed to spread my wings and try something new. I'd spent my entire life in the rural towns of Idaho and Eastern Washington. I wanted more. Hawaii sounded fun and exotic. I wanted to experience a different side of life.

"How can I become president if I don't go to a good college?" I said jokingly.

"I don't want you to go," she stated. She was adamant.

"I have to try," I said.

She never relented completely. In fact, she tried night and day to get me to stay.

The last weeks of high school were tinged with sadness, but I still found time for some fun and misadventure. One night, some of my football buddies came over when Mom was working an evening shift and I decided to cook spaghetti for us. As I waited for the pasta water to boil, I threw together a quick batch of tomato sauce, tossing in some onion, garlic, salt, and pepper. Of course, I was also generous with oregano, and as I pulled out the bottle and got ready to sprinkle it over my simmering concoction, one of my friends, Freddie, commented that it looked like I was adding "weed."

With that, he reached into his pocket and pulled out a bag of pot, suggesting that we substitute the oregano with our own special herb. I agreed, and Freddie poured a generous helping into the saucepan. We were all joking and congratulating ourselves on our creative new recipe, when my mom unexpectedly arrived.

"Mom, what are you doing here?" I blurted, as Freddie quickly shoved the empty bag down his pants. "You're not supposed to be home 'til seven," I reminded her.

"I got off early and thought I'd head home," Mom explained. "Oh, what a nice surprise: you're making dinner," she added. "I'm starving!"

My friend shot me a panicked look as I tried to discourage Mom from joining in the meal. I searched my imagination for an excuse. "Oh, this is no good," I tried. "We really messed it up. It tastes awful."

"Nonsense!" Mom replied. "I'm sure it's fine. I'll just doctor it up a bit."

"No, you don't want any of this, Mom," I insisted, but there was no stopping her. "Let me have a taste and decide for myself." My friends just shrugged and tried not to burst out laughing. I didn't know whether to laugh or cry or run away. "Hey, this isn't bad at all," Mom decided, giving our special sauce high marks. "You boys did a pretty good job!"

As I looked for a last-ditch way to protect Mom from "experiencing" our pot-laced spaghetti, I grabbed a small plate to serve Mom with the idea that I'd heap on the pasta and add the smallest dollop of sauce possible. No such luck. "C'mon Dwayne, don't be so stingy with the sauce," Mom ordered, grabbing the ladle from my hand. She proceeded to add a generous second helping of sauce and sat down to eat. Resigned to our fate, we served ourselves and joined her at the kitchen table. I ate a small amount, trying to offset whatever trouble I would soon find myself in. Someone would have to keep it together—or at least relatively together.

Within minutes, Mom had started giggling uncontrollably, and my friends joined in the raucous laughter. They were roaring so hard, I thought they might pee their pants. I was freaking out, but Mom was having a grand time, and she soon decided to serve herself seconds.

For the rest of the night, Mom told us crazy and inappropriate stories, punctuated with more hysterical laughter. My mother was as high as a kite, and my buddies, in a similar state, had no qualms about enjoying the ride with her. Years later I admitted to Mom that we had substituted marijuana for oregano, but she did not believe that she had actually gotten high. She would remain in denial—or at least refused to believe it—for the rest of her life.

On graduation day in June 1978, I stood in the hot sun on an open-air stage as the loudspeaker blared my name. Mom was sitting near the front, wearing the navy blue suit I'd bought for her so many years before with the dollar bills I'd earned from my trash removal job at the Arctic Circle. She was beaming. In truth, I'd never seen her look happier, more beautiful, or more proud. For me, she was the only one in the crowd.

After the hugging and congratulations, Mom quietly handed me a poem she had torn out of the local newspaper. It said everything she was thinking. I carried it with me until I was well into my forties even though, by then, it had practically disintegrated. I passed it on to my son as part of a video we made to celebrate his high school graduation:

> *My hands were busy through the day*
> *I didn't have much time to play*
> *the little games you asked me to—*
> *I didn't have much time for you.*
> *I'd wash your clothes, I'd sew and cook,*
> *but when you'd bring your picture book*
> *and ask me please to share your fun,*
> *I'd say "A little later, son."*
> *I'd tuck you in all safe at night*
> *and hear your prayers, turn out the light,*
> *then tip-toe softly to the door.*
> *I'd wish I stayed a minute more*
> *for life is short, the years rush past,*
> *a little boy grows up so fast.*
> *No longer is he at your side*
> *his precious secrets to confide.*
> *The picture books are put away*
> *there are no longer games to play.*
> *No goodnight kisses, no prayers to hear,*
> *that all belongs to yesteryear.*
> *My hands, once busy, are now still*
> *the days are long and hard to fill.*
> *I wish I could go back and do*
> *the little things you asked me to.*

Graduation made everything so real and final. As the poem Mom gave me said: "No goodnight kisses, no prayers to hear, that all belongs to yesteryear."

The fact that I was leaving had finally sunk in, and it had been decided that Mom would move in with Edweena in Spokane. She couldn't bear the thought of being alone in Walla Walla, and she would be a huge help to Edweena and her kids.

She had planned to quit her cooking job in the fall when I finally left for college, but her boss got wind of it and fired her on the spot. Desperate to raise cash to pay the travel costs to Hawaii, Mom and I both landed jobs that summer at the local Green Giant pea-canning factory. It was brutal, sweltering work. As fate would have it, I was in more of a supervisory role at the factory, while Mom toiled on the assembly line. She might have been tough and even selfish at times, but she was fiercely loyal and would bear any burden for her children. Her "sweat shop" job was just one more example of the lengths to which she would go to provide for me.

I remember one especially hot afternoon when I was making the rounds and noticed Mom from across the factory floor. She was working feverishly on the line, sweat pouring off of her face. She looked so hot and so exhausted that it pained me to look at her. I walked over to the assembly line to check on her. The floor was much too loud to have a conversation, but I grabbed a big fan from another station and set it up behind my mother. The workers glared at me, but I was the shift supervisor. "Don't even think about moving this," I warned no one in particular. How could I ever repay her sacrifices?

On one of our last shifts together, she pulled out one of my earplugs and shouted in my ear: "You're abandoning me, and it hurts."

I tried to tell her that I wasn't abandoning her. I could never do that. But there was so much noise on the factory floor that she couldn't hear, and though she could see that I was speaking, she didn't even bother to take out her own earplugs and listen. On the day I left, Mom drove me to the airport and walked me all the way to the boarding gate. We saw the plane sitting in the rain and watched the passengers scuttling up the metal staircase and disappearing inside.

I had never been on a plane by myself before. I was nervous about flying and I didn't want to leave my mother, but I was also excited about where the plane was taking me. For me, it was a beginning, not an end.

For Mom, however, this was her last child, her purpose, flying away. She'd do anything to postpone this moment. We stood there until the attendant made the last call for boarding.

"I have to go," I told her.

"Wait," Mom said and pulled something from her purse. "Here." She handed me a garish, heavy, gold-plated chain necklace holding a plaque with the message: *My son, the lawyer.*

Then she kissed me and hugged me and cried when I tried to pull away. The harder I pushed away, the tighter she squeezed. I finally relaxed and let her hug me. She kept squeezing until I thought I was going to burst.

"I'll be back for Christmas," I said as she finally released me, her teary face stained with mascara.

"I love you, my son. I love you."

"Mom," I said. "I love you too."

The wind and rain lashed me as I climbed the metal stairs. I turned back one last time and saw her smile bravely as she made the "I love you" sign—thumb, index and pinky fingers extended. I signed back to her and tried to turn away, but I couldn't until the attendant touched me on the shoulder. "We need to close the door now," she informed me. "You're the last one aboard."

It took all my strength to walk onto the plane without giving Mom a last look. As we took off into the sky I watched the world recede. I could see places I'd been, roads I'd driven, and as they all got smaller and smaller, I started to feel better.

The flight wasn't going to be the month-long sea voyage from India to the States that Mom had made at this same age, but there was the same promise of a new adventure awaiting me. I wanted to make the most of it. I wanted to make Mom proud.

WHO ARE YOU?

On one beautiful autumn afternoon, Edweena decided to bring Mom by my house. I had just finished a workout and was walking around outside when they pulled up.

Mom sat in the passenger seat, looking frightened and uncomfortable. Edweena powered down Mom's window so we could talk, but Mom recoiled as the glass descended into the car door, as if she'd never seen a power window work. At the sight of her darting eyes, I got a sinking feeling in my stomach.

"Hi Mom." I greeted her with a smile, hoping for the best.

She squinted at me but didn't reply.

Edweena came around to Mom's side of the car and stood next to me. "Mom, are you ready to get out of the car and come into the house?" she asked.

"Oh, I don't know," she started, but then her jaw went slack and a lost look came over her.

"Here," I said, and opened the door. "Let's get you out of there, get you moving."

I reached for Mom's hand, but she jerked away from me. "No! Don't do that!" she cried.

"It's okay, Mom. Here." She sat crooked and slouched in what looked to be an uncomfortable position. If nothing else, I wanted to help adjust her position so she could sit up straight. I gently reached under her arm to help prop her up.

"Nooooo! IT HURTS, YOU!"

I let her go and dropped to one knee beside her. "It's okay, Mom. You can just sit right there."

"That's right," she said.

Edweena leaned in close and said, "We'll just say hello and get going then." Edweena and I shrugged at each other.

"Who's that one?" Mom asked. I looked at her. She was pointing a shaky finger at Edweena.

"Edweena," I said.

"Oh," Mom said.

"Mom, do you know who this is?" my sister asked, indicating me.

I looked deeply into my mother's eyes, willing her to say my name. Her eyes were so far away, so empty. She had no idea who I was. Or if she did recognize me, she couldn't access the information. She'd already forgotten the question. She just blinked and searched my face with those empty eyes, looking for what?

"It's Dwayne," Edweena stated.

"Dwayne," Mom said. "Oh, yes, I'm so proud of him."

"It's me, Mom. Dwayne. I'm right here."

She smiled, and for a split second, I thought maybe she was joking with me. But no, she would never be that cruel. Only the disease is this cruel, delivering simultaneous jolts of sorrow, disbelief, betrayal, guilt. I dropped my head and stared at the ground. I wanted to cry right there, break down in huge, wracking sobs. Instead, I smiled as best I could and looked at her again.

She looked right at me, right through me. Was I just a strange face in the crowd? Was I someone she never knew until this very moment? I'll never know.

"He was such a wonderful boy," Mom said, looking directly into my eyes.

This was the day I had dreaded.

I averted my eyes, no longer able to look at this frail, confused woman, now squirming in pain. She continued speaking, but her words bunched together and came out as nonsense.

I feared that she was finally entering the final stage of Alzheimer's, when its victims lose their ability to remember family and their capacity to communicate disintegrates. Experts widely recognize it as the most difficult time, when the need for care becomes the most immediate and the severity of the symptoms are the most hurtful to the family caregiver. We knew this point would arrive, but how can you possibly be prepared for it?

"I don't know what's going on," Edweena said. "She was chatting nonstop just ten minutes ago. She was talking about India. She knew all the names of her brothers and sisters."

I didn't have an answer for her.

A breeze picked up. "Oh, that wind is cold," Mom stated, and even though it was a balmy day in the mid-eighties and the breeze was far from cold, hearing her strong, clear voice gave me the shred of hope that I needed.

Mom slouched a little more in her seat and I reached for her, afraid she might tilt sideways and fall out of the car.

"Here, Mom," I said as I propped her up.

She put a hand on my shoulder as I lifted her. My tee-shirt was damp with sweat from my workout, and she immediately drew her hand away and pulled a face.

"Get away from me, my son. You are all wet."

Relief welled in me as I heard her say, "My son." But it was a short respite. She continued speaking, but as before, it turned to gibberish. She looked at me, expecting a reply, so I shook my head and smiled, trying to muster a reassuring expression. She became very sad then and flinched away from me when I tried to touch her arm. I think, at some level, she realized that I couldn't understand her.

She seemed beaten, as we all were. I just wanted my mom back.

Edweena and I visited for fifteen minutes while Mom sat in the car and looked around. Sometimes, she appeared to be listening and added little comments like, "Oh really?" or "What's his name?" Sometimes the things she said made sense and sometimes they didn't.

Finally, it was time for them to go, and as Edweena got behind the wheel, I bent down to Mom's level to say goodbye.

"See you soon, Mom," I said.

She knitted her brow and shook her head in a gesture of confusion. Clearly, she didn't understand.

Just as the car began to pull away, I held our old sign, the hand signal for I love you, the one we'd used so many years before when I flew off to college and a new life. She was the one leaving now.

Mom hesitated for a moment, watching my hands and then recognizing the gesture. Slowly, as if raising a great weight, she lifted her hand to the window, showed me four fingers, and smiled. It wasn't quite right, but I knew that her intent was to convey her love.

I felt numb.

As I watched the car pull away down the street, I wondered what would happen next. I thought of the day I would get a phone call telling me she had been rushed to the hospital or that she'd died in her sleep.

And what about me? Would I be in her shoes one day, twenty or thirty years from now? I shook my head, pushing the possibility away. No way. Never. I didn't want to exist in a world where I didn't know my wife, my friends, my children, where the pieces of my life swirl about me like fireflies I could never hope to catch.

It was beyond my control. I could only hope that I didn't share Mom's fate.

MAY 2010
"HELLRAISER"

Mom turned eighty-seven years old.

There was no way to know how many birthdays she had left. Her age combined with her illness made each birthday feel like it might be her last. Each birthday now carried a weight that earlier ones didn't bear. It's not like it was possible to "make up" for not spending enough time together, not caring enough, or not doing enough. It was no longer possible to carry the day with lavish gifts or even a silly card. Those things didn't matter anymore— they couldn't. What mattered was how we celebrated. For me, her birthdays, along with special holidays, had become a second chance for the family to be present in the moment and spend quality time together.

It had been a process to get to this place of such simplicity and clarity. Each occasion became another marker and memory we would have after she was gone. Gift-giving itself had been stripped to the simplest acts and most basic values—providing small comforts for her and creating lasting memorials for us to remember her by.

Every year, the thought haunted us: Would this be her last birthday? Would she be with us for Thanksgiving? For Christmas?

I recalled how that mindset, that worry, had once led the entire family to do her birthday celebration up right. In pure Mom fashion, that meant going big, going glamorous. For her 80th birthday, less than a year after she'd been diagnosed with Alzheimer's, we took her to Las Vegas.

It was a fitting last hurrah that we all cherished, even if it challenged our coping skills. Mom loved to gamble and she loved Vegas. It was her kind of town, seemingly made to order: the gambling, the flashy clothes, the cheap buffets. You would have thought the demographic gods invented this town just for her. All her kids and grandkids were there to help her celebrate her birthday. Since Mom was already showing signs of dementia, we realized that this might be the last time we celebrated with her cognizant.

She played cards, she partied, she hugged and kissed us all with gleeful abandon.

Still, the signs of things to come were ever present. The second day we were there Mom started to have memory problems. We worried that it could be another mini-stroke, but Mom had blown us off and kept on going, back to the card tables and the roulette wheels.

Seven years later, Mom's birthday was far different, but no less important. We decided to make it a combination Mother's Day/birthday party, and once again, the entire family attended. My sister Linda coordinated all the food and invitations, and I hired a band to play at Mom's Aegis home.

Mom was sleeping most of the time now, waking up to eat but rarely for any other reason. But when we had the party, she stayed up for nearly two hours. My four-year-old grandson, Andre, kept going over to her and saying, "Hi GG." (GG is for great-grandmother.) She would look at Andre and make eye contact with him, as she would with me. You could see that something was spinning in her mind, but she just couldn't retrieve the thought.

The band played some of her old favorites, and the grandkids danced around. We all tried to enjoy ourselves and gave Mom gifts and cards. We were honoring the matriarch of our family. She couldn't talk but she was there. I wanted to believe that Mom really appreciated our efforts and all the attention.

Two years earlier, in celebration of her 85th birthday, we had a band play a special song we had composed and recorded in her honor. The song, performed by Seattle-based singers Ryan Smith and Jonathan Kingham, told the story of her life and was recorded in a "big band" lounge style, which we knew she'd enjoy and identify with on some level. Mom's song was appropriately titled "Hellraiser":

> *Hellraiser, couldn't hold me down*
> *Too much trouble for that sleepy little town.*
> *I wouldn't listen, still you believed*
> *Now it's all so clear to me.*
>
> *Where would I be without you?*
> *Without your love along the way?*
> *Where would I be without you?*
> *Tell me where would I be today?*
>
> *Stern, but forgiving, a fighter and a queen*
> *Daddy's girl, youngest of thirteen.*
> *You got by on nothing, so I could live my dreams*
> *Still you gave me everything.*
>
> *Where would I be without you?*
> *Without your love along the way?*
> *Where would I be without you?*
> *Tell me where would I be today?*
>
> *Hard times in the lines on your face*
> *Proof of what you made it through.*
> *Now I see you were always there for me.*
> *Now I'm here for you...*
>
> *Where would I be without you?*
> *Without your love along the way?*
> *Where would I be without you?*
> *Tell me where would I be today?*

Part 5.

Remembering and Letting Go: *Acceptance*

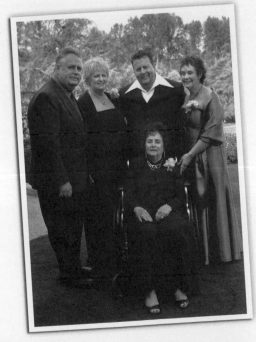

Masking the signs of Parkinson's at Dwayne's wedding,
2004: Larry, Edweena, Dwayne, Linda and Colleen

It was exactly how my mother
had described it. I could
easily imagine the scene more
than a half century earlier;
the colorful lights draped across
the courtyard; the American GIs
dancing with the well-heeled
ladies; the big band orchestra

image seemed
magical.
getting ready
realized that
's favorite
on the
It echoed
lobby
imagined my
these very halls,
to one of her
in her, later
day given that she'd smuggled
out of her dormitory, wrapped
around her waist as she
jumped the fence.
Maybe it was the fatigue
of the travel or the heat,
or everything from that day,
but I felt strange and
wonderful feeling in the
sun as the story played

India, circa 1934: A friend, Dennis Callahan (Colleen's brother) and Colleen

India 2008
Danny Boy

When I woke in my airplane seat, the first thing I felt was pain, shooting stabs, like electrical shocks in my legs and knees. It took a moment to focus through the fog and discomfort, before remembering that I was traveling to India with my wife for a vacation. We'd been in motion for thirty hours and were still hours from landing. I wanted to be unconscious again. If I had a parachute, I might have jumped.

Unsure of the time, I lifted the window shade, looked out the portal, and felt the pain, the discomfort, and the pressure in my head fall away as I gazed into the clouds and beyond.

The rising sun peeked over the horizon, illuminating the clouds with a deep red and orange glow. Below, spreading out as far as the eye could see were the mountaintops of the Himalayas, some so close that the fissures in the snow-capped peaks were revealed. It felt like something out of a dream, brilliant in its clarity and color, yet completely surreal, a blazing golden masterpiece, shifting with the light, filtering through the clouds. I'd never seen anything like it—truly, an awesome sight.

As I looked on, it occurred to me that somewhere down there, amid those mountains, Mom had gone to school, tutored—and tortured—by a cadre of strict nuns in white and black habits. I thought of her stories of those days and how she loved to hate the nuns and how much she had missed her dad and her childhood home.

I thought, too, that when she spoke of India, it was almost as if she were conjuring a dream, something that wasn't quite real, even to her. And yet, here I was, about to experience firsthand this land that had such an influence on her. The romance that India inspired was something she had passed to me; through her remembrances, I had inherited a passion for the exotic, a flair for the dramatic.

We finally landed and disembarked, and as I stepped into the cab that would take us to our hotel, I looked across the street to see a baboon looking back at me. He was in the median of the street, just staring at me.

The roads were impossibly crowded and there seemed to be almost no recognizable traffic pattern from street to street, with cars, scooters, and rickshaws mixing with a sea of pedestrians going in all different directions. Some were pushing carts, others were leading livestock, doing business, or just sitting and watching. I lost count of how many people perked up when they saw us, smiling and waving as we went by. And every time we pulled to a stop, a dozen beaming, beautiful children would rush our cab and tap on the windows, begging for change. Without fail, as we pulled away, they too would smile and wave at us.

We stayed at the Taj Mahal Hotel, a towering, beautiful building in the heart of Mumbai. (Sadly, the hotel today is known less for its luxury than for the deadly terrorist attacks that took place there six months after our stay; we watched in horror as news broadcasts showed flames shooting out from the windows of the very suite where Terese and I had stayed.)

Up until 1996, the vast city of Mumbai was known as Bombay, with the name originating from the Portuguese term for "good harbor." It's actually the second biggest city in the world, the commercial capital of India, and features the country's primary port.

We both "ooohed" and "aaahed" as we walked through the white domed lobby of the Taj Mahal Hotel, lined with artifacts, marble fountains, and amazingly detailed design work inlaid with gold. The people who worked at the hotel were generous and kind, almost to the point of seeming false. But their smiles and gestures radiated such an authentic warmth that we quickly fell under their spell.

Whenever I met someone new, or saw a sight, I couldn't help but think of my mother and how these same types of experiences must have shaped her as a young girl. We sat by the pool for awhile in the brutal heat and went for a walk as the sun set. There were monkeys playing in the distance, and I recalled Mom's childhood stories of exotic animals and elephant rides to town. Before going back to our room that day, we sat in the lobby and sipped on little glasses of coconut milk while Terese and I reflected on our day.

India was exactly how my mother had described it. I could easily imagine the scene more than a half century earlier: the colorful lights draped across the courtyard; the American G.I.'s dancing with the well-heeled ladies; the big band orchestra providing the soundtrack for the festivities. The image seemed so real it was magical.

As we were getting ready to go up to our room, I realized that "Danny Boy," Mom's favorite song, was playing on the hotel's stereo system. It echoed through the cavernous lobby atrium and I imagined my mom roaming these very halls on her way to one of her dances, dressed in her latest ball gown that she'd smuggled out of her dormitory, wrapped around her waist as she jumped the fence.

Maybe it was travel fatigue or the heat or the emotion of the day, but I felt a strange and wonderful feeling in the air as the song played on. Mom was there with me, at least in spirit and memory. I thought of her here with my future dad. I imagined her at her station during the war, tapping out messages in Morse code. I thought of her crooning "Danny Boy" to the ex-patriots in my grandmother's restaurant. What was it like for her all those years ago?

I was so compelled by the vision of my mom and dad dancing in that courtyard at the Taj Mahal that I later contacted my father to ask if he and Mom had even been there. While I rarely talked to my dad, I just had to know if my apparition had been real. Dad confirmed for me that, indeed, he and my mother had been to that very hotel, in that very courtyard, dancing the night away some sixty years earlier.

For the remainder of my journey in India, I felt as if my mother stayed at my side. I could hear her quip little comments and I remembered the stories she had told me as a boy. Once, when I saw a monkey on the street scratching at a mango, I recalled Mom telling me about a troupe of monkeys that lived in a tree outside her house and how she used to sit and watch them jump from limb to limb; she loved to sit there and watch them because, much of the time, they would watch her right back.

Another time, the day before we left, I witnessed a wedding in progress, a long procession of family and friends dressed in blazingly colorful clothes, dancing down the sidewalk, holding torches, shaking bells, beating drums, lighting firecrackers, and clapping. They were all singing at the top of their lungs, laughing and crying, completely unaware—or unconcerned—that people were staring. The groom swept his bride off her feet and twirled with her in his arms, around and around, causing the folds of her dress to wing out as they spun. I paused to watch, struck by their abandon, their sheer willingness to lose themselves in their celebration.

For a while afterwards, I couldn't stop thinking that Mom would have loved to have seen that wedding. A larger part of me, though, understood that she was already seeing it, that I am now my mother's eyes, that I carry the essence of her heart with me wherever I go. So as I walked on and left that scene, I took solace in the idea that Mom really was with me, not just in spirit, but in the most real and deep part of the person I am.

As we boarded the plane to return home, I was overcome with a feeling of sadness that I was leaving India. I had actually been looking forward to getting back, to sleeping in my own bed, to returning to a routine of work and family and friends. But I also felt as though I was leaving a riddle behind before it had been fully solved. The sights and sounds and smells of India are overwhelming and the mystery of the culture is ancient. I knew that in some ways—and certainly for a Westerner like me—India is impenetrable. But I still wanted more—more clues and more answers about who my mom really was. I felt as though I was leaving my heritage behind.

She had shown courage beyond belief when she left India and her family, but she was a woman who spent her life afraid of small things. She was fiercely independent yet constantly searching for the perfect companion, a man she couldn't have or, at least, couldn't keep. She laughed easily but there was also a part of her easily touched by depression and sadness. She worked hard for the things she believed in yet, at times, could be selfish and haughty. She lived with passion and exuberance, taking risks, but still harbored a terrible fear of dying.

Who was she? And how did this place help to shape her?

Later when I sat down with my journal to record the trip, my reflections were consumed by this dilemma: *Maybe I'll never have the answers I seek. Clearly, it's too late now for me to mine her for answers. That's the saddest part of all, isn't it? I'm writing this and referring to her in the past tense and yet she's still alive. She's still alive.*

DECEMBER 25, 2008
CHRISTMAS PRESENT

Christmas was always Mom's favorite time of the year. When I was a kid, the Christmas plans typically began the day after Thanksgiving and culminated in a grand party with an incredible meal, elaborate decorations, games, drink, music, and dancing. She made sure the season went perfectly, planning every last detail, right down to the song lists and the placement of the tinsel on the tree. These were the times I remember as being the happiest in her life.

She involved everyone in the actual cooking, and usually served at around four in the afternoon. There was a little taste of everything: Turkey, roast beef, mashed potatoes and gravy, sweet potatoes, green beans, sweet onions, big fresh rolls, and "green stuff"—the family's legendary pistachio pudding. "I only eat 'Tasty Food,'" she'd say over and over, like a mantra.

When we were stuffed to the gills, out would come the pies and cakes, and then it would be time to dance. Mom would drag each family member onto their feet and we'd stumble, bellies full, in time to the music, laughing all the while.

Today was my turn to host Christmas, and I've tried to keep the various traditions alive. Certainly, the decorations and the food retain the importance they've always had for us. I spent most of the day in the kitchen, getting everyone involved with the chopping, sauteeing, stuffing, and mixing. My son, Adam, showed up with Mom around noon and wheeled her into the kitchen

239

where she surveyed the hive of activity with a wide-eyed look of wonder.

"What happened here?" she asked.

"It's Christmas, Mom," I said.

Mom looked around the room. Terese was there, preparing a butternut squash soup. Adam had his son, Andre, in his arms. My daughter was there with her boyfriend, Ricky, along with half a dozen friends who'd stopped by to say hello. Frank Sinatra sang "The Little Drummer Boy" in the background.

"Bullshit," she stated. "I'd know if it were Christmas."

"It is so," I said.

I handed her a small tray of tea sandwiches I'd made especially for her.

"Nothing tastes good anymore," she said.

Although she was a lifelong lover of cuisines from around the world, nothing tasted the way it was supposed to anymore, and most of the time, what she did taste was overwhelming to her. Plus, it had gotten harder for her to swallow even small bites. Still, she had to eat. I was hoping the ritual of cooking and tasting our traditional "Tasty Food" would encourage her.

"Chips and dip," I said. "Your favorite. And if you don't tell me how it tastes, I won't know if we should serve it to the guests."

"I'll try," she said, like she was doing me a very big favor.

"Good," I said. "Finish that, and I'll put you to work."

Mom beamed and started to eat. After a few moments, she nodded approvingly. Mom was down to nearly 120 pounds by now, and any way we could get calories into her at this point was crucial. By including her in the cooking process and tapping into her desire to help, I knew I had a good chance of getting some food into her, and I was thankful to see her noshing away and enjoying the snack.

"I've had worse," she said.

We took a break to open presents soon after. When it was Mom's turn, we helped her unwrap her gift, a faux-fur blanket, incredibly soft. She raised it to her face, rubbed it along her cheek, and cooed softly. Then I wrapped it around her shoulders and neck and watched as her eyes rolled into the back of her head. She was in heaven. The joy of a comforting touch had replaced any desire she once had for jewelry or even nice clothes. Now it was only about the moment and the simple pleasure that emanates from a fleeting sensation.

In one sense, I found this to be terribly sad. She was no longer the person she once was. But, on the other hand, we are nothing if not creatures constantly changing, at the mercy of time and age. This was her lot and I was happy to be able to bring her some comfort, even if it was a case of "here one moment and forgotten the next."

It seemed like just a few Christmases ago that I had surprised Mom with a mink coat. We brought in this big box, and as she started to open it, I warned, "Be careful, it's alive." Mom reached into the box, felt the fur, and let out a scream as she kicked the box away. The sight of the fur and my warning had made her believe that there really was a live animal in that box.

Happily, it was a "gotcha" moment that Mom was still lucid enough to appreciate. Once she got over the initial shock, she relished her new fur coat, caressing it, and modeling it for everyone at the house. To her, that was the big-deal symbol that her son had really "made it." But those days were long behind us.

While we were opening presents on this Christmas, my grandson Andre, then two-and-a-half, helped provide us with a new

Mom memory. He was toddling around, going from person to person with a tiny, neon green-and-pink soccer ball. He would pick it up, drop it, and pick it up again. When he came close to Mom, she locked onto him and perked up. She reached for him and he responded to her, putting the ball in her hands. She looked at it, made a cooing sound, and then gave it back to him. He replied with a delighted chirp of his own.

"Ball," Andre said and handed it back to her.

"Ball," she replied and handed it back to him.

As I watched this exchange repeated, it came over me that this was the circle of life unfolding before my very eyes. Mom was now somewhere between a five and six on the Reisberg scale and the lucid moments she experienced were becoming shorter and more infrequent as the days went by.

As I watched my mother and her great-grandson passing a ball back and forth, I recalled Reisberg's other breakthrough determination: The degeneration of the mind under the influences of Alzheimer's mirrors the normal mental development of a child, only in reverse.

I saw that discovery playing out in my living room: These two human beings, linked by blood, yet separated by three generations and more than eighty years, were at the exact same place in the chain of cognitive development. Only one of them was at life's end while the other just getting started.

Once the gift giving was over, I hurried the party into the dining room. I knew that Mom would begin to get tired and nervous as the day wore on, so we sat down earlier than usual to eat. As we toasted the day, I could already see the window that connected us with "Mom" was closing. Just moments before we sat, she'd focused on a picture in our hall showing a wide vista and vivid wildflowers. She tried to reach for the flowers but, confronted by the picture frame, she became frustrated and suspicious. She suggested that something was wrong in the house, though she wasn't sure exactly what it was.

Now, at the table, Mom began looking even more agitated.

"That's it," she announced. "I'm done."

"But Mom, you only ate one bite. Try your mashed potatoes."

"I need to go," she insisted. "I need to go home to Edweena's. It's getting too late."

She was "sundowning," a term used to describe the irrational fear of the impending nighttime, a phobia that many Alzheimer's patients experience. Mom has been suffering from these episodes for some time now, and when one set in, her nervousness quickly segued to outright fear unless she got some reassurance that she was on her way home.

So we rose from the table, packed up her belongings, loaded her into the car (with a driver I had arranged for her), and sent her back to her Aegis home. Before she left, I kissed her on the cheek, told her I loved her, and wished her a Merry Christmas.

"Okay. Merry Christmas, my son," she said.

I stood there speechless, and before I could reply, she smiled her old sly smile. For a moment, the twinkle in her eye returned.

It was the best Christmas present I could have received.

I kissed her on the cheek again and closed the car door. As I watched the car slowly pull away, I could see that she'd retreated again—so quickly. The twinkle in her eye had been replaced by her fear of losing the light—she was not yet in her safe place.

When I started writing this book during the latter part of my mother's illness, I was sometimes gripped by fear and guilt, emotions that were fueled by my belief that Mom was dying a horrible death, that I couldn't help her, and that nothing has meaning when confronted with this cruel and unfair disease.

However, in that moment, when that bright soccer ball went between my mother and her great-grandson, I felt an unusual serenity come over me. For just that moment, I wondered if this disease is part of our natural lives, with its own hard lessons that remind us of what it means to be human.

We are all here for such a short time. Our lives are just fragile things. We spend so much time in the pursuit of our goals yet we are always traveling in a perfect circle. Just as an infant depends on her parents for everything at the beginning, so does the parent rely on their child at the end. It gives a person little solace, especially if they're spoon-feeding their infirm, confused parent or changing their diaper, but there is an element of nature involved in this process. That is something to celebrate or, at least, something to cling to in dark times.

Each of us has to look in the mirror every morning and prepare to live another day. We try to remind ourselves that we are lucky to have what we have for the time we have it. We are lucky to have our health, our families, our work, and our lives. And then there are our memories, those precious, private things that exist only for us. They are the only things we really have in this life. We have to cherish them in our time and pass them on as best we can.

GONE IS THE MOTHER I KNEW

Mom had been hanging on for so long that I lived in constant anxiety of the phone call I knew was coming—probably sooner rather than later. It wasn't an entirely irrational fear, but it was made worse by the fact that the fear of losing her had haunted me all my life. As a kid, I would have awful nightmares in which Mom would somehow disappear; I would wake up terrorized that she might actually be gone forever from my life. I would thrash myself to a sitting position and then slowly blink awake to the realization that she was in the next room, still here, through my heart continued to pound wildly, unable to catch up with the sense of relief that now flowed through my bloodstream. She was all I had then, and I couldn't imagine living without her.

Ironically, that emotion seemed to intensify as she slipped farther into the grip of dementia. Even though she couldn't communicate with me and didn't recognize me, there was still so much I needed from her. I was not unselfish enough to tell her: "Okay Mom, I am releasing you now to a better place." Even though so much of what made her Mom to me was no longer available, I just couldn't let go. I didn't want to lose my mother.

The "close calls" have been coming more frequently, but when the phone range one April evening, I really believed this was it, the one I had been dreading for so long.

Kathy, the executive director of Mom's Aegis community, was on the other end. I felt terror rising in my throat. She had phoned me before with an emergency situation involving Mom, but this time her voice didn't have its usual sturdy and reassuring tone. "Dwayne, you'd better come down here. Your mom is unconscious, but breathing. The paramedics are just arriving."

Fortunately, I was close by. In less than two minutes, I raced into the Aegis parking lot and made a mad dash for the entrance. Mom was in her room, pale and unresponsive, the paramedics already at work trying to revive her.

As I moved in and bent close to her, I could see that she was barely breathing. I yelled in her ear, and her eyes cracked just a bit. This is it, I thought. *I'm losing my mom.* She was dying right in front of my eyes.

As the paramedics prepared to transport her to the nearby hospital, her eyes fluttered open. I saw utter sadness peering back out at me. She looked like a frightened deer, her pleading eyes for just a moment locking onto mine. It was if she was looking at me and saying, "Help me, help me." What could I do? Nothing. At that point I was equally helpless.

I called my sister Linda and she said she would meet me in the emergency room. Then I called Edweena, three hundred miles away in Spokane, and told her I'd keep her updated. The hospital was only two blocks from the Aegis community, but still I arrived ahead of the ambulance and waited for what seemed like an eternity. My thoughts ran wild. *Where could they be? What is taking so long? Maybe Mom didn't make it. Is the hospital staff just preparing how best to tell me my mother is dead?* A hundred scenarios ran through my head—all bad.

Linda arrived at some point, and shortly thereafter, a staff member finally came out to inform us that Mom had arrived. She was alive and stable. The doctor had ordered intravenous fluids, and with the added hydration she had begun to come back. Linda and I were taken to her room. Relieved, I sat down and put my iPhone up to her ear to play an Etta James song, "Cadillac." She gradually opened her eyes and gave the slightest hint of a smile. I breathed out, as though I had been holding my breath. I had not lost her just yet. She was here still. Physically, at least.

As I watched my mother, I tried not to ponder what was yet to come or how I've seen others suffer from this disease in our Aegis communities. Instead, I rifled through my memories and pulled out my favorites: her smile, her laugh, her jokes, the way she hugged me, all the little things that made her so unique and alive. I tried desperately to hold onto those images, to go back and reside in those happier times, but I couldn't quite get past her current condition: frightened, confused, alone.

Who is this person? I asked myself. *She looks like my mom, although much more frail and tired. But she's a stranger to me. Where is the interaction, the conversation, the teasing? Where are the mannerisms that I know so well? Could this really be my mother, the woman who worried about me constantly, who was there every time I needed her, who spent a lifetime building me up and making me the man I am today?*

Finally, I turned away from my thoughts and back to her. Mom's chest under the sheets was rising and falling, her breathing steady now, normal. I looked again at her face and found her staring right back, more through me, though, than at me, as if I were an apparition. *This is my mother,* I reminded myself. *Gone is her laugh, gone are her devilish ways, gone is her swagger, but this is my mother. This is my mother.*

THE CIRCLE OF LIFE

My daughter, Ashley, got married on a beautiful June day. It was the moment of my lifetime, hers too, of course. But as my sisters and I spent time with her that morning, Ashley was more worried about her grandmother.

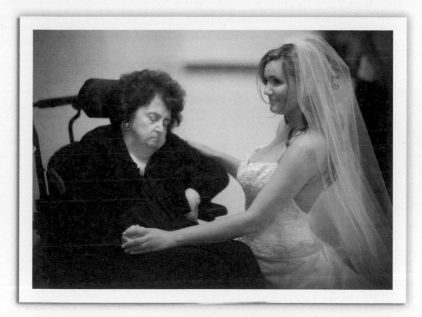

Ashley (Clark) Rea's wedding 2010 with grandmother, Colleen

"When is Gram coming?" she asked Edweena. Ashley and my mother were extremely close. Both were romantics, and in their times together over the years, they had plotted and planned and dreamt of this special day. When Edweena explained that Gram was too ill to attend, Ashley took it badly. So although we were only hours away from the ceremony, my sisters made special arrangements to have my mother attend Ashley's wedding.

Moments before I was to walk my daughter down the aisle, Gram was wheeled into the dressing area. Ashley's eyes lit up. Adorned in her white wedding dress, she kneeled down and hugged my mother, telling her this was the moment they had talked about for over twenty years. Having her grandmother there made the wedding complete for Ashley, and it filled me with overwhelming emotion and joy. We all felt so lucky that, despite her condition, Mom could be present for this and so many other family milestones and memories.

A few days later, with Ashley's wedding day still fresh in my mind, I went to visit Mom with my four-year-old grandson, Andre, in tow. She was back at Aegis, having recovered from her hospital ordeal in April, though she had received a new diagnosis, the Cheyne-Stokes condition, an abnormal pattern of breathing.

When we entered the facility, we found her in the lobby, sitting in her wheelchair at a table with some other residents. She was sleeping, her mouth agape. I wheeled her to a quiet corner of the lobby so Andre and I could visit with her in private.

Even with the movement, her eyes remained closed and I was concerned that her breathing seems so labored, even though it fit perfectly the Cheyne-Stokes pattern. She would almost gasp for breath, followed by a short exhale, then nothing for few seconds, and then take another big gasp for air.

I studied her face and assessed her body. Her arms were still bruised from being poked and prodded with needles and IV treatments during her hospital stay in April. Andre noticed her arms and rubbed the bruises, saying "GG has an owie, Papi."

"Yes, Dre," I explained. "Be very gentle with GG, she's tired and hurting."

Sensing that this was a person who needed some love, Dre stood on his tiptoes, grabbed my mother's head, and pulled it toward his face to give her a kiss. "Careful, Dre, GG is sick." He continued to softly pat her arm and bruises. Despite her condition, Dre loved his great-grandmother, and he instinctively, poetically, gave her all the love and tenderness he had.

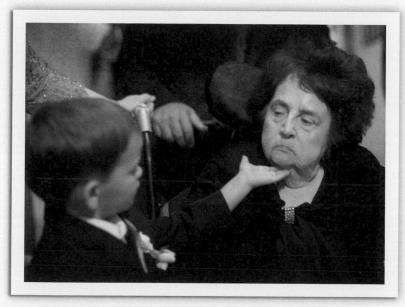

Andre Clark and Colleen, June 2010. Ashley's Wedding

Still, his actions didn't disturb her, and so I tried more forcefully to wake her up. "Mom, are you tired?" I asked. No response. "Mom, can you open your eyes?" Still no response. I made one-way small talk with her. "Mom, your hair looks nice today. Who did your makeup? I like it very much. You look like you have lost weight," I added, trying to resort back to the humor of years past. I even tried calling her by her childhood name to jar some sense of recognition: "Collu, are you in there?" Nothing.

I recalled how she used to ask us, beg us, not to let her die, to keep her alive using whatever means necessary. *Is this what she would have wanted, sitting here in a hallway, unable to interact, unable to recognize her own family, struggling to get out each and every single breath?*

I couldn't answer that question. And even if she'd wanted to, she couldn't answer it for herself; she was no longer even aware that she was alive. In that moment, I know I didn't want to continue my role in her request. I suddenly felt an understanding of why some people had chosen to help their suffering family members end their lives. *Was death a more merciful option?* As I sat there listening to my mother's laborious breathing, I thought, in this instance, it probably was.

My mother wasn't asking me to do anything. She couldn't, of course. So what could I do?

I thought about a conversation that my friend Lem and I had a few years earlier about his mom. She had been in and out of the hospital for months. She nearly died on one occasion and she got mad when the doctors brought her back. Shortly thereafter, she told Lem she was ready to go. He told me, "Dwayne, at that point, I had to make peace with her and tell her that we'd all be okay—I told my mom that she could leave this planet and move on. I was releasing her," Lem continued. "She died two days later."

As I mulled that conversation, it suddenly occurred to me: Was Mom hanging on for us? Did she actually want to move on, but couldn't because she was worried about her children?

I moved closer to her so she could hear me as I whispered these words: "Mom, I know this is a very hard time for you. You have been a fabulous mother and guide for me and for all your children. I have always loved and adored you. All that I am I owe to you. You have given me the incredible gift of confidence, which allowed me to become successful. You taught me how to love my kids more than life itself. You always stood by me, bad behavior or good. I know how much you want to take care of your family, but I know how hard your condition must be for you. I want you to know that it is okay to move forward, to leave this world and to go on to the next. I will love you forever and I will see you in due time and we will be together again. We will all be fine, Mom. I love you so much."

I completely surprised myself with this impromptu speech. Never in a million years did I think I would ever give my mom "permission" to go, but I believe that was what she needed to hear. I didn't know if Mom would live another two days or another two years. But I think I gave her some peace that day.

Finally, as my grandson and I were leaving the building, an ambulance sped by with sirens blaring. Without missing a beat, Andre, with typical four-year-old candor, stated, "I think that is for GG."

Not today Dre. Not today.

The Last Gift

I've heard comedians joke that hospitals are no place for sick people; they're certainly not for elderly residents with end-stage dementia. Hospitals are designed for acute issues; they're simply not equipped to provide the loving care a frail, sick person needs in their last days.

In what would become her final weeks, Mom was, unfortunately, in and out of the hospital. Her doctor tried to impress on us adult children that it was time to take stock and reconsider our approach. He spoke to me privately and told me in no uncertain terms that we were punishing my mother with treatment. He expressed his belief that the time had come to put her into hospice care.

Although there could be two, three, even as many as four transitions to hospice and back to Aegis, at least our mother would get comfort rather than painful treatments that weren't going to change the outcome. Life in a hospital is not relaxing and nurturing—it's 24/7 of poking and prodding, lights and noise. In his stern but caring way, the doctor said it was time for relief, not more frantic trips to the ER.

My sisters didn't want to give up; they wanted to keep fighting the good fight. But somehow in our exhaustion, the transition to hospice became a reality, setting the course for our final journey with Mom.

By July, the main challenge we had with Mom was that she had developed a huge hiatal hernia that hindered her ability to process food. When she swallowed, she was prone to aspirate her food, which could choke her or cause pneumonia. After dinner, someone would have to keep her up for two to three hours to allow the food to process properly. My sisters had started visiting even more, and Sally continued to come in to sit with Mom and help in the afternoons. They all fed her and advocated for her and loved her as best they could.

I took a short vacation in the middle of these touch-and-go summer months, never being quite sure if I should put everything on hold, or continue living my life. *What makes sense, what will enable me to live with myself more?* I wondered.

The fall was fast approaching. Terese and I had planned an exotic, two-week trip to Turkey, Jordan, and Israel. It was difficult making the decision to be away, but we determined that it would be okay, that our lives shouldn't be put on hold indefinitely. I needed to explain to Mom where I was going and I felt the need to say goodbye—just in case.

So I made a special visit on October 9. I told her for a second time that it was okay for her to go, but this time I selfishly asked her to please hang on a little while longer, to not pass away until after I got back. "If you have to leave now, I understand, but I'd like to be here to say goodbye to you." Both scenarios allowed me to think of myself as loving; either way, I hoped she saw me as a good son.

The next day, Terese and I left for Jordan. The trip was wonderful and I only called home a few times. Mom remained stable, and it seemed like she was given a timely reprieve.

We returned from Turkey on a Friday night, October 23, ready for a weekend of recovery from jet lag. The next morning, on finding the kitchen essentially devoid of the basics, including coffee, I volunteered to go to the grocery store. I was in the market when I finally got the call I'd been dreading.

Mom was worse than she'd ever been. Mom was dying. This time it was real. I could feel it.

Linda called the priest to give her last rites. We all pitched in to call other family members and our closest friends. About twenty people collected at her bedside. By then, she was struggling to breathe, her gasps quick and shallow. By Monday, two days later, her respiratory rate had slowed substantially, which for someone in Mom's condition is usually a sign that the end is likely to come quickly. Morphine would make it easier on her, but it was out of the question as she was allergic to the narcotic and it could actually make her feel more pain.

As aggrieved as I felt watching her suffer, I was also gratified that Mom had "waited" for me, provided me with one last gift, one that I both wanted—and needed. I got the sense that deep in her being, she remembered who I was and cared about everything we'd try to do for her. It was a selfish thought, a rationalization, perhaps, but I needed that bit of acknowledgment.

The moment I had feared since I was a little boy was finally upon me. I was sobbing, holding her head in my hands as I lowered my cheek next to hers and whispered: "Mom, I know you're leaving. Thanks for everything you've done for me. I want you to be comfortable, and you'll have a joyous after-life."

At 7:50 a.m. on October 26, 2010, my mother, Mary Colleen Callahan Clark, passed away. She was eighty-seven years old and had lived with dementia for nearly one-tenth of her life.

Goodbye

I'd long thought about my mom's funeral and what it would be like. Just like the self-help exercise in so many books, I'd trace out the steps in my head. I'd wonder who would come, what would be said, and how I'd handle myself throughout the day.

Now, with Mom really gone, I wanted to improve upon my musings and create the perfect service with the right readings, speeches, music. I sat down and wrote the eulogy I would give and even put together a video montage; I poured my heart into both, hoping to provide a moving, appropriate tribute to my mother, showing who she had really been and what she had meant to her family and friends.

Apparently, though, I was missing the mark. The day before the funeral, Mom came to me in a dream. She stood right in front of me, lecturing me as if I were still a boy back in Lewiston. In language illustrating that, like the nuns in India, the after-life could not completely tame her wild ways, she told me what she thought of my efforts: *Do not put that video out there. That shit is not me. Let ME talk.*

I woke with a start and spent the next twelve hours almost revamping the video practically from scratch—my mother's spirit guiding me as I added back some of the rough edges and allowed her true "unedited" character to shine through. This was the woman we knew and the person we admired for her unpolished, raw honesty and her simple enjoyment of whatever the day would bring.

Never in my wildest fantasy did I dream her funeral would turn out to be as festive as it was. My mother was a private person, and despite her outlandish ways, she wasn't one to share her "dirty laundry." She didn't gossip, she didn't have a circle of confidantes that can be so typical of single women of a certain age. Her best friends were her children and grandchildren.

In her earliest years, of course, Mom had plenty of friends and acquaintances; for the most part, everyone who met her loved her, and she could strike up a conversation with just about anyone, affectionately referring to them as "honey" and treating them like a life-long friend.

That had changed with, first, the divorce and, then, aging and Alzheimer's. In the last forty years of her life, she really had no one. Maybe she'd spend time with the occasional boyfriend (who she usually outlived), but no one close. Her best friends were her children and her grandchildren.

So you can imagine my surprise when over two hundred people showed up for her service on October 29, 2010.

We never asked anyone to substitute a charitable contribution in lieu of flowers, because my mother would have wanted the flowers. She got them too—over eighty arrangements. The priest said he had never seen so many flowers in one place.

I was so proud of my family that day. All of my siblings were present. My niece Tiffany and grandniece Dylan sang a beautiful rendition of "Ava Maria," one of Mom's favorite hymns. My nephew Ryan and my son, Adam, made me so proud as they spoke with great love and affection for their grandmother. My daughter, Ashley, did a reading, and one of the most profound memories was when Alex, my thirteen-year-old great-nephew, bravely stood up in front of this large audience and gave an incredible reading, struggling mightily to honor his great-grandmother and speak for his generation. Then it was my turn. My tears were flowing as I approached the podium, a lump in my throat that felt as big as a softball.

Thanks to my years as a CEO of a mid-sized corporation, I am used to and comfortable with speaking in front of large audiences, but giving your mother's eulogy makes it a completely different task. I didn't just want to relay some information and break the ice. And I didn't just want to give the usual platitude-laden eulogy. What I really wanted to do was to make them laugh, to know or recall the funny side of Mom, the side that said whatever she pleased to whomever she pleased, never standing on ceremony. I started with an anecdote about Mom and actually dropped the "F" bomb in church. People laughed, but I could tell they were stunned. I explained, for anyone who hadn't seen this colorful side of her, how swearing was her way of responding, of surviving really, whenever something threw her off balance. It was an integral part of her personality, and to me, on that day, it felt altogether appropriate, right even, to bring a bit of her spirit to her final celebration.

And so I laced my talk with a few more curse words, recalling how refreshing it was to be around Mom and that salty, direct way she had of speaking her mind. In a politically correct era when people verbally tiptoe through conversations, as if walking across a field of mines, my mother would lace up her boots of profanity and nonchalantly hop, skip, and jump through that same field. If a situation was full of shit, or she didn't give a shit, or the food tasted like shit, she'd say so. It was embarrassing and it was refreshing. It was Mom.

I didn't want to be crude for the sake of it, but as I explained to the priest after the service, "I felt it was more important to be true to Mom than respectful to the church." He laughed and said that maybe more people would come to mass if he talked like I did during my eulogy.

As we left the church, the bagpipes played and the drums beat, the "good-looking" men in their kilts making the kind of music my mother had been raised on and loved.

I knew exactly what Mom would say. "What, all this for me? Well, don't let it stop."

When everyone was outside we released a hundred white balloons with her picture on them. It was one more fitting moment of celebration for her fun-loving spirit. We watched those balloons float up into the sky for a long time, almost watching her take the last ride of her life, with all of us practically envious of her high-flying act. For the little kids at the funeral, we told them that the balloons were actually GG going to heaven, and they smiled at the simple thought.

I was not nearly so sanguine in the days immediately following Mom's funeral. It was as if I had come down with a spiritual and emotional flu, letting all the anger, fear, worry, and loss fully infect my soul. Away from others, I finally let myself feel the full effect of those emotions.

Terese and I kept things simple, going to the grocery store, eating comforting meals at home and her listening to me recall those teenage years as the man of the house doing a hodge-podge of homemaking, yard work, and bill paying. All the simple tasks that were giving me comfort now. Funnily, it was as if my mom was more present now than she'd been in the last couple of years. I felt her by my side as I slowly came out of my grief.

It was when we got home from one of our trips to the market that I had the eeriest sensation that my mother really was going to stick around.

Terese and I were bringing in our shopping bags from the car, and as I set mine on the large island in the middle of our kitchen, I saw a white balloon poking up on the underside of the counter. It was one of the balloons we'd made for her funeral, but I didn't remember any of them being saved. We'd released all of them into the sky as our last celebration and remembrance.

And yet here "she" was, bobbing along in front of me and then bouncing to my favorite chair in the sitting area by the window. I was too freaked out to put the groceries away or do anything normal—she was staring at me, or her photo was, and following me around.

Terese was seeing what I was seeing and she had no idea where the balloon came from either, or what was making it float and move about. We even went looking for open windows to see if there was a draft.

Well, our search provided no answers to the mystery. The only thing I knew for sure was that Mom was having the last laugh, and I thought of her smiling down on all of us.

Part 6:

What I Learned:
Advice for the Journey

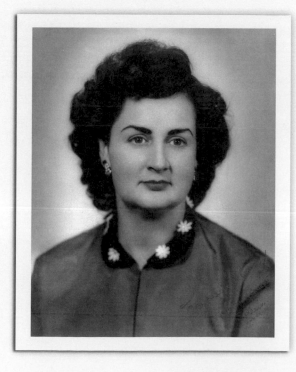

Mary Colleen Callahan Clark, circa 1943

LOVE All Trust few, Always
paddle your own canoe.
"Quote"
that's what Mom always
used to say. As her son,
it's my job to _____
thin _____
_____ _____
the _____
our _____
shar _____
occ _____
to _____
wha_____
to

One of Colleen's famous Christmas photos. Colleen, 1999

Advice to Use and Pass On

Intellectually, we know that aging is part of life, but Alzheimer's is a disease that can challenge—and even break—the closest friends and family of someone who suffers from it.

If anyone should have been prepared for my mother's disease, it should have been me. I've spent almost my entire professional life devoted to services and communities that care for the elderly, and I've seen all of the difficulties and challenges that patients and their families contend with. But I wasn't prepared—not by a long shot. And throughout my mother's ordeal, I came to the realization that no one ever is. Intellectually, we know that getting older, getting sick or frail, getting dementia, or even getting Alzheimer's is a part of life. It's not until someone we love—someone we care for and are responsible for—is gradually pulled away from us by the disease that the reality sinks into our hearts and souls.

It is natural—and very normal—for family members of a person experiencing dementia and Alzheimer's symptoms to deny that possibility for as long as possible and to attempt to maintain the ordinariness of "regular" life. Yet, facing this disease and getting through and beyond denial provides huge benefits for everyone—better medical care, leading to better quality of life for the patient and family members, better caretaking of the patient and support for loved ones, and better insight to ease the challenges and create more opportunities for closeness and closure.

When I look back at my story and the journey I've been on as a son and as a professional, I tried to think about what would be most helpful to others. What practical lessons and advice could I share that would make a difference? To-do lists aren't what most of us need. We need to-be lists, to-allow lists, to-know lists, to-accept lists. That's what will help us Alzheimer's families get through as best as we possibly can.

As I thought about what was most helpful to me and what makes the biggest difference with families at Aegis, I realized that understanding is the most powerful thing. When we truly understand what's happening and what will help, it makes our personal choices and decisions much easier. Understanding comes over time, through bits of wisdom, practical medical insights, health strategies, emotional preparations, and support mechanisms that can improve things as much as possible and give us comfort along the way.

So what I've come up with are Fourteen Guidelines for the Journey, a series of stepping stones to help you find your way. This may not be all-inclusive for everyone dealing with Alzheimer's, but they helped me and my family as we sought to cope, understand, and find meaning and acceptance—and they had a positive impact on my mother's care and well-being.

First, though, I want to share the gift of the most memorable pieces of advice I received while my mom was sick. These are words and messages that doctors, caregivers, and other family members provided, and so I wrote them down and then returned to them over and over at times when the disease became harder to bear. This is advice I've since passed on to many others along the way. Highlight the ones that resonate with you and tape them above your desk or dresser or tuck a copy into your wallet so you can read them when you most need to.

- Understand from the outset that things will not improve.

- Ask for and accept help.

- Try to be easy on yourself. This may well be the most difficult thing you'll ever do.

- Try not to feel guilty. None of this is your fault.

- Fill your heart and mind with good things.

- Sometimes, with the afflicted person, comfort is the only victory.

- Remember that you're not supposed to get everything right.

- This time will pass and you will have the memory of how you responded to the challenge.

- When it's time, put away your grief or anger or disappointments and live your life. That's what your parent, grandparent, or spouse would have wanted.

- Take time for yourself to meditate, to walk alone, to sit in silence, and to breathe—and breathe deeply.

- *Love all, trust few, always paddle your own canoe.*

The latter is what my mother always used to say. As her son, it's my job to carry that message forward. Now, though, I think she'd appreciate this added sentiment: *But even though we are all paddling our own canoe, we all share the same vast ocean of water, trying to make the most of what we are given, trying to find our own truth.*

Fourteen Guidelines for the Journey

1. Information Is Healing

We get information in all kinds of ways, and they all support our ability to make sense of the challenges in our lives and in the decisions we face. We get information through:

- real-life stories (like this book) and conversations with friends

- experience as we live, deal with events, and shift in our thinking, feeling, and actual physical responses to a situation

- researching books, articles, Websites, lectures, and classes

- intuition, spiritual sources, and the unconscious mind

There are numerous books, videos, organizations, and support groups available and consulting a variety of sources can be particularly clarifying and empowering for anyone coping with Alzheimer's. As such, family members and caregivers should actively seek a deep level of knowledge and understanding as early on as possible—and update that research over time. This will help you (and other family members) fully grasp the mental and physical implications for the victim of this disease, but it will also help you realize the journey that you have embarked on as well.

You will have the tools and knowledge you need to recognize what will be a new kind of normal: the agitation, the paranoia, the phobias, the memory loss. You will understand that your loved one now has memory gaps and will feel and display frustration, even rage, when they can't verbalize their thoughts or recall faces and memories. The person wants to hold onto their identity, and the communication and processing skills necessary to do so, but the disease is getting worse. As a caregiver, you will feel like perhaps you are losing your own mind too, "going crazy." That's why knowledge of what to expect early on is so critical; knowing what is normal at different stages and what to expect in the future will help assuage any feelings of guilt that may surface and provide much-needed emotional comfort and assurance as you move forward.

ORGANIZATIONS

Alzheimer's Association

The national Alzheimer's Association provides information about Alzheimer's disease, resources, research advances, publications, and events. www.alz.org

National Parkinson Foundation

This organization provides information about Parkinson's disease, online tests for tremor and clinical depression, "Ask the Doctor" forums, and other resources. www.parkinson.org

BOOKS

The 36-Hour Day: A Family Guide to Caring for Persons with Alzheimer Disease, Other Dementias, and Memory Loss in Later Life, by Nancy L. Mace and Peter V. Rabins, Warner Books, revised edition, April 2001. This classic guidebook for families and caregivers offers informative insights and clear, specific, and realistic advice.

A Dignified Life: The Best Friends Approach to Alzheimer's Care, by Virginia Bell and David Troxel, HCI, 2002. A presentation of a model of care for Alzheimer's patients, stressing empathy and friendship, for nurses, adult day center staff, and families of patients.

Don't Toss My Memories in the Trash: A Step by Step Guide to Helping Seniors Downsize, Organize, and Move, by Vickie Dellaquila, Mountain Publishing, 2007 An experienced professional organizer and senior move manager shares valuable tips on downsizing and moving for both seniors and their family members.

Alzheimer's Early Stages: First Steps for Family, Friends and Caregivers, 2nd Edition, by Daniel Kuhn, MSW, Hunter House, 2003. With the advent of earlier diagnosis, this is a much-needed book on the early stages of Alzheimer's to help families cope. It includes an excellent resource section.

Dementia Beyond Drugs: Changing the Culture of Care, by G. Allen Power, M.D., Health Professions Press, 2010. An excellent and provocative recent book about drugs and dementia that advocates away from using psychotropic drugs and the importance of environment, behavior, and activities.

Still Alice, by Lisa Genova, Pocket Books, 2009. This award-winning *New York Times* bestseller is a beautifully written, heartbreaking novel about the devastating effect of Alzheimer's disease, told from the point of view of an Alzheimer's sufferer named Alice.

VIDEOS

"Why Do They Do That?" by Teepa Snow. A poignant, engaging, and sometimes funny two-hour workshop for family and professional caregivers explaining the complexity of Alzheimer's and memory loss and its impact on the brain and the person who suffers from the disease. It also provides practical ways to interact, help, and connect. The video can be obtained at www. AegisLiving.com.

"The Alzheimer's Project." This four-part documentary hosted by Maria Shriver can be viewed online at www.hbo.com/alzheimers and is available as a three-CD set at Amazon.com and other retailers. A presentation of HBO Documentary Films and the National Institute on Aging, the video includes cutting-edge research, interviews with individuals at various stages of the disease, and the experiences of caregivers.

2. USE A PHYSICIAN SPECIALIZING IN AGING— AND FIND THE BEST

Many older people have had the same internist or general practitioner for twenty or thirty years. They've developed trust in and familiarity with that person and commonly resist turning over their care to someone new—a veritable stranger by their standards. Yet geriatricians, neurologists with a specialty in memory loss, and other doctors with specialties in aging can provide a much higher level of care. They understand the many forms and diagnoses of memory loss, including Alzheimer's disease and Parkinson's, the challenges of nutrition, and the range of treatments and protocols needed to deal with the loss of abilities such as speech and swallowing. Finding the right physician can extend your loved one's life by two to five years—and improve the quality of their life.

There are challenges to finding a qualified physician. To begin with, there is a shortage of geriatricians, and some of these limit the number of Medicaid patients they accept into their practice. Ask for referrals through organizations and your health insurance provider. Consider "best doctor" listings provided by trusted journalistic sources that you can search for on the Internet. Depending on your access to specialists in your community, consider an initial consultation for a treatment plan with preferred physicians. Even if they are based farther away, he or she can at least act as a specialized consultant to your local doctor.

When is the right time to make the transition? It's rarely "too soon." When you begin having questions about your loved one's health, care, and memory, that is usually the best indication that the time has come to seek out the expertise of a physician trained in elder medicine.

3. UNDERSTAND THE DISEASE

Many people "know" something is wrong for months and even years before they seek—and get—an official diagnosis of Alzheimer's disease. In truth, Alzheimer's is a diagnosis of symptoms, as there is no definitive test that documents the disease.

A diagnosis is avoided, delayed, or missed altogether for a number of reasons: 1) Many of the signs of the disease run parallel to the natural aging process, including memory loss, struggle for words, forgetfulness, and perhaps new anxieties, confusion, or neediness; and 2) there doesn't seem to be any "good" that comes from the diagnosis, though there can be treatments that substantially slow the disease process.

While it is natural for us as human beings to forget things as we age—our brain cells actually begin deteriorating in our early twenties and we all forget where we left our car keys from time to time—it is the repetitive and continued loss of familiar things that should concern us, especially when it interferes with our daily schedule, plans, and relationships.

In the beginning, when we start to see our loved one "getting older" or "declining," it's hard, even impossible, to know if they're experiencing normal aging, an illness that can be treated, or a degenerative disease that can be improved with certain types of care. Our resistance and fears, coupled with the older person's desire to see themselves as "just fine," can keep us from taking actions that will be beneficial and helpful for everyone—and can lead to a much higher quality life. Weight loss, poor nutrition (especially in earlier stages), and depression are co-existing diagnoses, all of which can be managed and even overcome.

Understanding brain function and Alzheimer's

Our brains are superconductors of information. Every second, billions of neurotransmissions, tiny electrical impulses containing messages, travel from one brain cell to another. Electrical and chemical neurotransmitters allow these messages to travel across tiny gaps between the neurons. Alzheimer's causes the network to break down by inhibiting the brain's production of acetylcholine, a chemical that essentially lubricates the brain at the microscopic level. Without this lubricant, a sticky plaque forms and limits the flow of information. In addition, protein fibers within the neurons become twisted and tangled, further diminishing the ability of brain cells to communicate with each other. As a result, memories are lost, behavior changes, and the personality that you associate with the individual eventually disappears.

Although many people lump all memory loss under the umbrella of Alzheimer's disease, there are many different types of memory loss diseases. Huntington's disease, for example, is an inherited brain disorder that destroys brain cells and affects a person's cognitive and physical abilities, but doesn't show until a sufferer is in their thirties and early forties. Parkinson's disease, though sometimes confused with Alzheimer's, is a degenerative disorder of the central nervous system that impairs the muscles.

Dementia, from the Latin *de* (without) and *mentia* (mind), and a term first used to describe Roman soldiers who had sustained head injuries on the battlefield, is another loss of cognitive brain function that is often associated with Alzheimer's, though it can result from other diseases as well. Dementia symptoms in those suffering from Alzheimer's can manifest differently from person to person. The most prevalent, though, include mood changes, loss of problem-solving skills, difficulty communicating, disorientation, change in personality, and the appearance of new behaviors.

THE 7 STAGES OF THE REISBERG SCALE

In 1982, Dr. Barry Reisberg published a 7-stage scale of Alzheimer's disease that is used to this day to help assess the disease's progression in individuals. Stage 1 is no impairment. Stage 2 is typical of normal aging and the "senior" moments so many middle-aged people experience. Stages 3, 4, and 5 show progressive impairments in a person's ability to remember, plan, organize, and take care of themselves, with slow declines sometimes followed by precipitous and shocking drops in functioning over the course of days or weeks. The person may start something—like cooking a meal—and never finish it—or may have trouble keeping track of their household. Memory aids like notes and reminders may help. There are many ways the disease presents itself as it becomes manifest in this middle period of the disease. Stereotypes are just that—they may or may not reflect any individual's symptoms. Stages 6 and 7 refer to the late stages of the disease where the person is literally disappearing mentally and needs intensive and, ultimately, complete physical care.

GENERAL SIGNS

Some of the more obvious signs of Alzheimer's are difficulty finding the right words. Forgetting that a loved one has passed away and speaking of them as if they are still alive may be common. Short-term memory is quickly affected. You may ask them what they had for lunch the day before and they may not be able to tell you.

A person may show changes in behavior and personality, becoming belligerent, loud, flamboyant, or uncooperative. It may feel as if they are just letting their true personality out, or they may be uncharacteristically aggressive, paranoid, or compulsive. Their brain has a drive to fill in information—even if it's made up. The person's self-protective psychology pushes them to cover up.

A Red Flag: The Transient Ischemic Attack (TIA)

A TIA, sometimes referred to as a mini-stroke, can be a red flag for declining health and the risk of developing Alzheimer's. These so-called "warning strokes" produce stroke-like symptoms such as sudden confusion, dizziness, loss of balance, or numbness of the face, arm, or leg. TIAs occur when a blood clot temporarily clogs an artery and part of the brain doesn't get the blood it needs. Most TIAs last less than five minutes and do not cause permanent injury to the brain. To some people, TIAs can seem so minor that they do not get medical treatment afterward, but they are extremely important indicators or predictors of a major stroke or Alzheimer's, and potential clues to other brain or arterial changes that should be evaluated by specialists.

Other Coexisting Signs

Alcohol use and excessive drinking can co-occur with Alzheimer's and be a way for a person to cover up and ease their anxieties, although it can also be a cause of weaker cognitive function. This complex and hard-to-address scenario should be discussed with the professionals you're working with.

Depression and other symptoms and medical conditions should be definitively evaluated and treated to enhance quality of life and as clues for diagnosis. There can be many complications due to multiple medications, side effects, and co-occurring conditions that can affect the health of an older person, but are easy to overlook or not to recognize.

4. Watch, Observe, and Journal

Behavior analysis is the only way to diagnose Alzheimer's and to plan the best care and environment to support a person once they've been diagnosed. Family members play a crucial role here and keeping a journal of symptoms and changes can be enormously helpful—I know that it was for me.

As soon as you start noticing changes in condition, jot down the dates, what happened, and what's out of the ordinary. It could be eating, breathing, weight gain or loss, or behavior changes such as hiding things or displaying inappropriate anger. These notes will provide data for a person's decline or improvement.

For example, my mother was originally diagnosed with Alzheimer's and later her Parkinson's was identified. When we put her on Parkinson's medication, for about six months she actually improved. She gained weight, she started walking and talking, and the Parkinson's "mask" went away. We wouldn't have had that detailed knowledge if we hadn't written observations down. Remarks like "her face got frozen," on a particular date were helpful for physicians to create treatment plans.

A journal also helps give you a marker of where a person is in the progression of Alzheimer's disease. When a person stops talking or eating, you can see where that falls on the Reisberg scale. The average life span after a person is diagnosed with Alzheimer's is seven years. When my mother reached the final stage at the age of eighty-seven, we knew she was very near the end of her life, and we were able to mark occasions and involve our extended family and friends in a way that felt healing and meaningful for all of us.

5. Look for Love and Understanding When Choosing a Care Facility

I know when I meet new friends and the topic of my business comes up, the response is usually, "My mom would never live in a place like that." This is when I ask, "Like what?" It seems like most people's impression of assisted living facilities hasn't changed from the stereotype: the sterile, smelly place where people wander around aimlessly and yell in the hallways. When I show them photos of our Aegis communities, the response is always the same: "Wow, I never knew that places like this existed."

There are many options like Aegis today—places of warmth, caring, and professionalism. Once a family or person with memory loss raises the question of needing help or starts discussing a change in living arrangements, that is the best time to take steps to find more care from an assisted living community. No one ever says, "I did this too soon."

The emotions are wrenching, but once the initial decision is made, there are straightforward steps and options to consider, and the process usually goes very quickly and with less struggle than the months that preceded it. If there's been a crisis that precipitates the transition to assisted living, you will find very supportive help and information through the Alzheimer's Association and many agencies in your area.

When that moment arrives, how do you choose? How do you imagine what's right, when nothing seems right about the situation at all? There are five factors to consider:

- Type and size of the community and level of care

- Location

- Reputation

- Costs

- And most of all, love and understanding—what is the connection between staff and residents and your sense of their understanding and caring?

Every state has different licensing terms and regulations and there are some thirty to fifty licensing categories across the United States, but basically there are four tiers of communities: mom-and-pop homes; assisted living communities with widely different models and levels of services; nursing homes; and the hybrid continuum-of-care retirement communities.

The smaller, private mom-and-pop residences usually have five to six residents and are often located in a converted private home. The owners or managers can be quite good—and sometimes not so good—but the training and level of care may be unsophisticated. Sometimes staff sleeps at night so it's possible for a resident to have falls from bed or other problems that won't be checked or discovered until morning. These homes can be very convenient and affordable, and there may or may not be a lot of understanding, but the expertise will definitely be limited.

The assisted living model requires that staff members are licensed and that someone will be "on their feet" 24 hours a day. The quality and style of assisted living communities vary as much as motel and hotel rooms do. You've got the basic Motel 6 model, the high-end Four Seasons model, and everything in between.

Nursing homes refer to facilities' focus on having skilled nursing available 24 hours a day. However, only about 20 percent of the elderly who are frail need skilled nursing. Most of the care that is needed can be provided in an assisted living or mom-and-pop community. Help with daily living such as bathing, medications, eating, and general support do not require skilled nursing. A skilled nursing facility is needed for residents with complicated conditions, for example, a patient who is on dialysis, recovering from surgery, and dealing with other serious situations.

Recent years have seen the rise of continuum-of-care retirement communities. These are communities that are designed for active residents by providing them with plenty of opportunity to golf, shop, and engage in social events and other activities; later, they have the option to transition into assisted living, if the need arises.

It's important to balance location, convenience, care, oversight, and the relatives who will be most available for visiting with the type of care and the community that feels right to you and your family. A wonderful community that isn't accessible isn't ideal nor is a nearby home that feels sad and where residents don't seem loved and valued.

Reputation is essential, as are your own observations. When you begin talking to friends, neighbors, doctors, and local organizations, you'll be amazed at how much expertise there is out there and how much personal experience people have with the different communities. When you begin to take steps, you'll find that a wealth of very helpful information will be made available to you.

And you can supplement those recommendations with an inquiry to your local Long-Term Care Ombudsman Program or by visiting their National Resource Center at www.ltcombudsman. org. The ombudsmen serve as advocates for seniors and their families and regularly visit and monitor care facilities. Another great resource is your state's licensing agency for assisted living. State inspectors conduct in-person annual inspections of each assisted living community and write up written reports of their findings that you can access.

Costs are a very real concern, but as a close friend and colleague says, "You do not want to negotiate with your heart surgeon." For the most part, higher costs equate to a higher level of service and a higher ratio of staff to residents. On the cost issue, I recommend, to the extent it's possible, to look for the right fit before looking at "cheaper" or "budget" options. You may be surprised at the resources available to you through insurance, savings, Medicare, and Medicaid that can make your community of choice possible. To discuss the financial plan for assisted living, you can meet with the marketing director at the community you're considering and you can get information and guidance through the sign-up process.

All of these essential practical issues aside, the basic advice I give to anyone is to look for love and understanding. It may sound silly, but seek out places where you see people hugging residents. See if the residents appear to be clean and look at their nails, teeth, and clothing. If you visit a place where a resident has food remnants on their clothing or their nails are dirty and untrimmed, you know the care probably isn't what it should be. Visit at both quiet and active times of day, like lunch. You'll see the residents and how they're cared for and how they are treated at meal times. Is spilled food cleaned up? Are the staff members making conversation with the residents, or are they abrupt? Are they loving, and do they address people by their name? Do they know the residents' priorities—for example, their favorite foods, a little bit of their personal history, or a topic they like to discuss? A place may not be beautifully up-to-date, but if you feel that the residents are receiving caring attention, that is worth a lot.

Love and understanding go a long way. The care is incomplete without emotional nurturing.

6. LIVE WITH THEM IN THE DISEASE

When a person has Alzheimer's, a lot of what they do doesn't make sense. We don't "get" how their misfiring brain is creating the different and confusing person in front of us. It's so typical of us as family members to say things like, "Mom, you know your sister died years ago," or "You know Uncle Kenny doesn't live with us anymore." So often, even knowing better, we try to argue with the person who is losing their mind to dementia. This is called "reality therapy," and it is not effective or useful.

All it does is agitate the patient. Their brain is telling them that a person is alive. It used to be that professionals would try to reorient the person to the correct time and place, but we now know this is very harmful because it frustrates the person and leads them to think you are lying to them. With paranoia a part of the constellation of Alzheimer's symptoms, these confrontations over the "truth" play into that tendency. The patient's trust factor goes way down, making everything more challenging.

The important thing to remember is that if you live with the person in their reality, there can be much more harmony and connection. That's why Aegis communities have life-skills stations, where, for example, we display vintage clothes, typewriters, and rotary phones. Many of our communities have "bus stops" where residents can sit on a bench to get "going to work," before their memory lapses and they move on. And our residents love the antique cars we have in some of our community outdoor areas; one, for example, has a 1946 Buick in the parking lot, which brings back so many memories. Some residents view the community car as their own, one they can wash, gas up, and drive, just like they used to, though, of course, the cars don't actually start or go anywhere.

These are all examples of ways to accept and live with our loved ones in their reality. It minimizes the agitation and allows for whatever connections that do exist to come forward.

7. CREATE FAMILIARITY AND COMFORT

If you were going to move to a 300-square-foot room tomorrow, what are the ten things you'd absolutely miss if you didn't have? It could be a chair or picture you love. Other people want yarn and knitting needles, a musical instrument, photo albums, or books about travel. If someone is religious, a crucifix or a Star of David often gives comfort and connects the person with deep memories from childhood. It is important to make sure that you allow Alzheimer's sufferers to retain whatever items provide them with real joy or passion.

Sometimes the biggest victory is giving the person comfort—especially when we try to celebrate and discover that old traditions like parties or dinners or brunches are too stimulating and stressful. Consider adding decorations to the room that recall great memories, such as a picture of winning an award or a video from a family occasion or certain music that is a reminder of some special time or event—these are all ideal ways to create comfort and familiarity.

With my own mom, for example, because it was very hard for her to put on lace-up shoes, I bought her sock-shoes that were easy to slip on and really warm. She loved them. I bought her several cashmere and silk blankets and other items that felt good on her skin. Especially in the late stages of the disease, these small comforts are all you can do, and they are quite powerful—much more so than you might think.

8. HONOR AND CELEBRATE

During the late phases of the disease, traditional ways of celebrating and honoring a person can be overwhelming or simply impossible. Yet honoring the person is so meaningful for us and for them.

In our family, we would have family gatherings in my mother's room for birthdays and holidays, sometimes with ten or even twenty people squeezed in. We would reminisce, telling stories like, "Mom, remember when we did?" Or, "Remember the time we went to Disneyland?" Or, "Remember when you broke your foot?" We'd have an actual conversation with her, assuming that she was present and listening, even if she was, emotionally, far away from us in the moment.

There's a tribute aspect to that type of storytelling and there's a residual benefit. It helps the family with closure and is healing in its own right. It speaks to the sufferer's life, to their character, to who they were as a person. Bringing out stories and memories and connecting with other family members in the room all elevate the person beyond their disease. At the darkest hour, this is a very important thing to do. We get beyond seeing just the physicality of the person, who is now ninety-five pounds and weeping. We get beyond watching the decline and crash of a person who at one time took up so much emotional and psychic space in our lives.

The person wants to be remembered differently, and we want to remember them differently. When we honor and celebrate and give tribute, we create an opportunity for that to happen.

9. MAXIMIZE THE CALORIES

As Americans we want people to eat a certain way. I once wrote a blog about a ninety-two-year-old woman who was eating sugar packets from the table. Her family was horrified and called her doctor to ask what they should do.

The doctor's advice? "She's ninety-two. Let her eat the sugar packets!"

Obviously, no one's going to let a resident drink a bottle of bourbon or eat ice cream by the gallon, but in the later stages of the disease, calories become more important than nutrition. The ability to eat declines as the body's functioning declines, and the person just needs nutrition of any type. I would bring my mom carrot cake with icing an inch high, French fries, and other enticing, easy-to-eat goodies. It would provide comfort, familiarity, and calories. You can try to tempt an Alzheimer's patient with special high-nutrient meals of, say, crisp green salad or fresh red beets, but come on! It's not going to happen. Go for the calories. All of you will be happier and—ironically—the patient will probably be healthier.

10. TRANSPORT AND CONNECT WITH MUSIC

Music has incredible therapeutic value. First, there's an almost instinctual physical response. For example, when you put on upbeat music, or a favorite rock and roll song, your body reacts and you start bouncing in your seat, moving your head, and getting a smile on your face. The music physiologically changes your body and attitude. Music itself can construct different moods, and it increases blood circulation. It can be comforting also because music inspires powerful mental associations. Our bodies and hearts "remember" if you will, specific songs, such as a lullaby from childhood or the music played during a couple's first wedding dance.

In my mother's case, we found that music—soft, low in tone, and slow—also helped her to fall asleep at night and sleep longer hours. In the daytime, when we wanted to encourage her presence and alertness, we'd put on her favorite big band music and dance with her. It would often get a big smile out of her and also increased her overall alertness.

In every way, music has such a therapeutic value that it's extremely important to make it a part of your loved one's day.

11. Awaken with Nature

It's critical for people with dementia to spend time outdoors. even if they're living in a more urban environment. Even prisoners are mandated to be outdoors for one hour a day! Unfortunately, people who suffer from Alzheimer's are too often relegated to their rooms or the halls of their community.

Anthropologists tell us that we're hard-wired to respond to nature and that there are universal environmental factors that make us feel good, such as water, sun, shade, and natural light. This concept is known as biophilia. When we're cut off from nature we suffer. By contrast, if you undergo surgery and are exposed to natural light through a window (versus a brick wall), your body will heal faster.

Though it's difficult to get them out of their beds or other comfort zones, people with Alzheimer's need to go outside and experience nature's stimuli for healing and comfort—the feel of rain drops, a breeze on the skin, the warmth of the sun, the chirping of birds, the smell of recently cut grass. Even the sounds of children playing or an airplane passing overhead can have a positive effect.

These sensations stimulate memories and experiences that make a person feel more whole and alive. I remember taking my mom out to pick flowers. She always loved the smell, so I put one bud up to her nose and she sniffed it very softly and surprised me with an audible "Ahhh." Even though she wasn't talking a lot, there was some kind of reaction. Her sensory system said, "I like that," as it also did the fresh air and the sun beating on her face. At Aegis, we've even designed clear umbrellas so residents can go outside even if it's raining to get vitamin D, oxygenate their bodies, and still enjoy and experience all the sights and sensory pleasures of the Great Outdoors.

12. GIVE THE GIFT OF TOUCH

Touch is an incredible healing mechanism, so we can't forget to touch the person with Alzheimer's, in spite of their bad breath, messy eating, and lack of responsiveness. More than that, we need a specialized plan to incorporate touch into their lives. Touch is a primal need, as classic studies and Dr. Ashley Montagu's pioneering work showed more than twenty-five years ago. Without touch, research shows, people and animals fail to thrive.

Touch comes in many forms and can fill the void of lost relationships. There is massage, Reiki, and healing touch. At Aegis, we've had success with reflexology because sometimes a traditional massage can irritate an elderly person's fragile skin and even cause it to tear. Reflexology actually stimulates vital organs and parts of the body through touch of the feet and hands. A wonderful way to experience the power of touch is with a gentle scalp massage during a hair shampoo. Pets can also provide a healing touch and intimacy. My mom thought dogs had their place up until she was seventy-five years old, and then all of a sudden she loved dogs. They were on her lap and kissing her and giving her something she physically needed.

So touch is a major element that can provide comfort, care, understanding, and stimulation. Discover ways to bring touch into your loved one's life, and it will ease both of you enormously.

13. ALWAYS REMEMBER DIGNITY

One thing I want this book to promote is that every person deserves dignity. We may lose our cognitive functioning and our personality may change, but we don't lose our humanness.

Even though a person with Alzheimer's is stuck in their private world, disconnected in many ways from their loved ones, we shouldn't take away their dignity.

That sense of dignity can manifest in a variety of ways. For instance, my mom would never go out of the house without her hair fixed and lipstick applied. So even when she was bedridden, we made sure her hair, face, and nails were done. My mom was always a snazzy dresser, so even at the end, we tried to keep nice, clean, presentable clothes on her. Another woman may have never cared about makeup or clothes, but perhaps she would find it degrading to be bathed by a male nurse; let your care community know and make sure they are following your instructions.

You are displaying real honor towards a loved one and helping them retain their dignity when you do for them what they would want to do for themselves and in the way they would want those things done.

We can measure ourselves and the care we're giving and providing by the honor and respect our family members are shown. Dignity, even in the end, is worth so much.

14. Get Care for Yourself and Others

Family members often fall into caretaking roles depending on their inherent personalities, the quality of their relationship with the person with Alzheimer's, and practical issues like work, family, and location. The caregiver who takes on the greatest daily responsibilities is a heroic person.

According to dementia expert Teepa Snow, caregiving is not an option for many people—it's not something you may feel equipped to do or equipped to do for a particular person (which was the case for Snow's own mother when her grandfather developed Alzheimer's during her childhood). You have to be able to live with and accept the person's reality and allow it to be.

Even the most giving, skilled, and loving family caregiver can get overwhelmed rather quickly. To be an effective caregiver, you have to start with caring for yourself—you need to know when your trouble light is about to go on and say: "WARNING, TAKING A BREAK."

Caregiver burnout has become rampant in today's society, as people who are compelled by their desire to be a great caregiver usually don't give into their own needs. The end result is bad. The caregiver's physical and mental health condition deteriorates; and the person receiving the care also ends up getting substandard care because the caregiver doesn't have the resources to do a good job.

So watch for the warning signs: Are you tired, not getting enough sleep, or being awakened in the middle of the night to do care duties? Do you find yourself irritable and getting angry and resentful with the person you are caring for? Are you having trouble completing normal tasks, like cooking, shopping, or doing household chores? If so, your warning light is flashing brightly.

The most important, essential thing you must do for yourself is to make sure you get sleep. If your sleep is frequently interrupted by demands from your loved one or from your own piled-up work, personal needs, or worry, you may need to get help. Home health care agencies can provide nighttime caregivers. Some local government agencies can provide assistance if you don't have the funds. Other resources are local assisted living communities that often offer respite-stay programs. Take a break, even for a week, and move the person you are caring for to a respite program just so you can get a physical and mental rest and recharge your batteries. Do this as often as you need to.

There is no guilt in trying to take care of yourself. We all have to accept that we are mortal, that we have needs, and that in the end we can't help others if we don't also help ourselves.

Perhaps we all need to be reminded of the lesson I learned making potato soup with my mother, about being gentle with ourselves and with others. We may think we can do and do and do. We may believe we have somehow failed if we haven't done enough, when there isn't "enough" for a person with Alzheimer's. We may need to remember—over and over again—to be kind to ourselves and to each other. We are all doing the best we can.

Sending you positive energy,

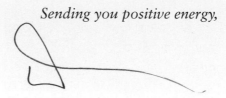

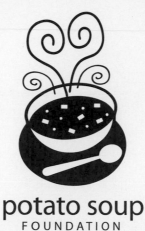

potato soup
FOUNDATION

ALL OF THE PROFITS FROM THIS
BOOK ARE BEING DONATED TO THE
POTATO SOUP FOUNDATION AND
THE ALZHEIMER'S ASSOCIATION.

When Dwayne Clark was a teenager, there was a time when he and his working mother had no money and no food. This forced the two to get creative. One night they "borrowed" some potatoes and made enough potato soup to last for a week. This experience was life-changing for Dwayne and gave him the drive to create a thriving senior living company known as Aegis Living.

During this week of severe hardship, Dwayne and his mother, Colleen, avoided any sense of despondency by focusing on the future, imagining all that Dwayne could be when he grew up. Like his mom, Dwayne was a dreamer with all kinds of grand ideas. But that week, his mother and their temporary misfortune taught him that even the hardest working people can find themselves in desperate situations. "Don't ever forget this," she admonished him, holding a spoonful of soup between them. "This is very important to remember. Always remember."

Then she gave him some practical advice that would stick with him for the rest of his life:

"If you ever have people working for you, treat them like family, support them, and help them when they need it because things don't always work out for people. They probably won't ask you for help or tell you their troubles, but you can tell when things aren't right for people if you just pay attention to them. Be there for your people and they will always be there for you."

That advice became the foundation of Dwayne's business philosophy when, decades later, he founded Aegis Living. Today, his mother's heartfelt advice doesn't just inform the company's day-to-day operations. In 2005, Dwayne and Aegis Living established a not-for-profit, tax-exempt organization called the Potato Soup Foundation: Its principle purpose is to help Aegis employees and their families during times of tragedy and extreme need.

The Foundation has since provided members of the Aegis "family" with emergency medical treatment, emergency housing, funeral expenses, and a variety of other financial and emotional aid required by crisis situations.

If you would like to donate to the Potato Soup Foundation, please send your contribution to:

> The Potato Soup Foundation
> 17602 NE Union Hill Road
> Redmond, WA 98052